ScrubTales™ Nurse Practitioner

A Real-World Career Guide That Tells the Truth About Responsibility, Identity, and Clinical Decision-Making

ScrubTales™ Series 1 — Core Clinical Careers

Mason Preddy

MMP
MASON MAISON
PUBLISHING™
REWRITING THE NARRATIVE
MASONMAISON.PUB

MASON MAISON
PUBLISHING™
REWRITING THE NARRATIVE
MASONMAISON.PUB

Copyright and Disclaimer

This book is intended for informational and educational purposes only. It is not medical, legal, financial, or professional advice, and it does not replace consultation with licensed professionals, accrediting bodies, employers, educational institutions, or regulatory agencies.

Healthcare careers vary widely by state, country, institution, specialty, and time. Scope of practice, certification requirements, compensation, benefits, job availability, and working conditions may change. Readers are responsible for verifying all requirements, credentials, and regulations applicable to their individual circumstances.

The author makes no guarantees regarding employment outcomes, income, career satisfaction, or professional success. Any examples or scenarios described are illustrative and should not be interpreted as promises or predictions.

By reading this book, you acknowledge that all career decisions are your own responsibility.

Chapter 1

Dedication

This book is dedicated to **Joanna Robertson, DNP, FNP-BC, PMHNP** — whose voice, clinical wisdom, and deep respect for the inner lives of clinicians helped inspire **Anna Remedy, DNP, FNP-BC, PMHNP**, and whose work continues to model what sustainable, humane practice can look like in modern healthcare.

And to the **Beachfront Gals** — for the laughter that restores, the honesty that grounds, and the constant reminder that a meaningful career is allowed to coexist with joy, friendship, and a life well lived.

You each embody the quiet truth at the heart of this book: alignment is not indulgence — it is survival.

Chapter 2
Welcome

Becoming a Nurse Practitioner isn't simply the next step in nursing. It is a structural shift in responsibility, identity, and daily emotional load.

This book exists because too many people enter the Nurse Practitioner role with excellent intentions—but incomplete information. They are told what the role *can* be, what it *allows*, and what it *means on paper*. They are rarely told what the role *feels like* over time, how the responsibility accumulates, or how the cognitive and emotional demands change once decisions become yours to own.

ScrubTales™ Nurse Practitioner is not a motivational guide, a scope-of-practice manual, or a checklist for advancement. It is a lived-reality system designed to help you decide—honestly and without pressure—whether the Nurse Practitioner path fits who you are, how you're wired, and what you need to sustain a long career in healthcare.

This book is written for:

- Registered nurses actively considering the Nurse Practitioner path
- Students exploring advanced practice roles
- Early-career Nurse Practitioners seeking clarity and recalibration
- Experienced clinicians reassessing fit, longevity, or next moves

You do not need to read this book quickly. In fact, you shouldn't.

ScrubTales™ is built to be used deliberately. Each section is designed to slow you down at the exact moments where rushed decisions often lead to regret—before school, before debt, before identity lock-in, and before responsibility compounds.

At the center of this book is a simple principle:

Fit matters more than capability.

Many people *can* become Nurse Practitioners. Fewer should.

That is not a judgment. It is an invitation to clarity.

As you move through this book, you will encounter emotional tolls, real workdays, hard questions, financial realities, negotiation boundaries, and early-career stabilization strategies. None of these sections exist to persuade you toward or away from this role. They exist to protect you from choosing a path that contradicts who you are.

This book will ask you to be honest—with yourself most of all.

If you proceed thoughtfully, the decision you make at the end—yes, no, or not yet—will be one you can stand behind.

Chapter 3

How to Use This Book

This is not a book meant to be read once and shelved.

ScrubTales™ Nurse Practitioner is designed to be returned to at decision points—sometimes quietly, sometimes urgently—when the questions you are asking have shifted or sharpened. You may choose to read it straight through, beginning to end, absorbing the full arc of the role before making a decision. You may also open it selectively, turning directly to the section that speaks to the pressure you are feeling most acutely right now.

Both approaches are valid. Both reflect different moments in a longer decision-making process.

If you are deciding whether to become a Nurse Practitioner, begin with **The Toll Booth** and **Day-in-the-Life**. These sections are designed to reveal what the role *demands*, not just what it allows. They show how responsibility, pace, and expectation surface in ordinary workdays, rather than idealized descriptions or promotional narratives.

If you are already on the path—or questioning whether to continue—move directly to **Before You Commit™**, **Fit Check™ (Mini SCRUB*fit*™)**, and **Next Moves™ — Not Every Pivot Is an Exit**. These sections exist for moments when momentum alone is no longer enough to answer the questions you are carrying.

If financial pressure is shaping your decision, **Financial Landscape™**, including **The Long Payback**, is designed to provide clarity without hype—showing tradeoffs, timelines, and constraints rather than promises.

This book is meant to be used, not admired. It is not structured for passive consumption. Highlight it. Skip sections. Return later with new eyes. Let your reading pattern reflect where you are, not where you think you should be.

The goal is not reassurance.

The goal is alignment.

About (gl)

Throughout this book, you'll occasionally see **(gl)** next to a word or phrase. That tag simply means the term is included in the **Glossary** at the back of the book. Healthcare has its own language, and the goal of these tags is to reduce confusion, build vocabulary over time, and keep you moving without having to stop and Google every other sentence. If you see **(gl)**, you can keep reading and circle back later—or flip to the glossary right then if you want the definition in plain English.

Chapter 4
Why This Book Exists

The Nurse Practitioner role is often described in terms of autonomy, authority, and opportunity. Those descriptions are not wrong—but they are incomplete.

They explain what the role enables: expanded scope, increased decision-making power, professional advancement. What they rarely address is what the role requires from the person inside it.

Becoming a Nurse Practitioner is a shift into sustained responsibility. You are expected to assess, decide, explain, and stand behind decisions—often with limited time, imperfect information, and competing pressures. That responsibility does not arrive all at once. It accumulates quietly, patient by patient, encounter by encounter, until it becomes part of the background of your professional life.

Over time, the work stops feeling episodic and starts feeling continuous.

Some people experience that weight as clarifying. It sharpens focus, deepens purpose, and brings coherence to their professional identity. Others experience it as exhausting—not suddenly, and not catastrophically, but through the steady depletion of cognitive and emotional reserves.

That difference is rarely about intelligence or ability.

It is about fit.

This book exists to help you understand which outcome is more likely for you *before* the cost becomes personal, financial, or irreversible.

Chapter 5

Who This Book Is For (and Who It Isn't)

This book is written for nurses considering advanced practice, students deciding whether the Nurse Practitioner path truly fits, early-career Nurse Practitioners seeking clarity, and experienced clinicians who find themselves quietly questioning sustainability.

It is for people who want to understand not only whether they *can* do this work, but whether they want to live inside it over time.

It is not a scope-of-practice manual, a program directory, or a motivational speech. It will not promise fulfillment, income, prestige, or balance. It does not exist to sell the role or to dissuade you from it.

Instead, it offers something more useful: an honest picture of what this role feels like to live inside—day after day—once the title is real and the responsibility is yours.

Chapter 6

A Note on Alignment, Responsibility, and Choice

Choosing a healthcare career is not about proving capability. Most people considering this path are already capable.

The more difficult question is whether a role can be sustained without gradually eroding the parts of yourself that matter outside of work.

Alignment does not mean ease. It does not mean the absence of stress, challenge, or sacrifice. It means fit. It means that the demands of the role align closely enough with how you think, decide, recover, and carry responsibility that the work remains viable over time.

This book respects your intelligence and your agency. It does not tell you what you should choose.

The decision is yours.

The information is here to support it.

Chapter 7
The Toll Booth

Every healthcare role has a cost of entry.

For Nurse Practitioners, that cost is not paid all at once.

It is collected gradually—decision by decision, patient by patient—often so quietly that you don't notice the toll until you've already passed through.

The Nurse Practitioner role changes the *nature* of responsibility. As a Registered Nurse, responsibility is shared, distributed across protocols, teams, and hierarchies. As a Nurse Practitioner, responsibility consolidates. You are expected to assess, decide, explain, and stand behind those decisions—sometimes immediately, sometimes later, and sometimes long after the encounter is over.

The toll is not simply stress. It is sustained cognitive load.

You carry differential diagnoses in the background of your thinking while moving through your day. You weigh risk while managing time pressure. You reconcile clinical judgment with documentation requirements, organizational constraints, and patient expectations that do not always align. Even when a shift ends, unresolved questions often linger—not because you missed something, but because medicine rarely offers clean closure.

This is the first toll: **decision ownership**.

Over time, decision ownership reshapes how you experience work. Encounters stop feeling discrete. The work becomes continuous. One decision informs the next. One compromise creates another. You are not just reacting—you are anticipating, preventing, explaining, and revisiting.

For some people, this feels grounding. The responsibility sharpens focus. It brings coherence and professional identity into alignment. For others, the same responsibility creates a low-grade, persistent drain—one that doesn't announce itself as burnout, but slowly erodes energy, patience, and emotional reserve.

The difference is not talent.

It is tolerance for sustained responsibility.

There is a second toll that often goes unnamed: **visibility**.

As a Nurse Practitioner, your decisions are visible in ways that extend beyond the patient encounter. Charts are reviewed. Outcomes are tracked. Complaints, if they arise, attach to your name. Praise does too—but visibility is rarely neutral. It adds a layer of self-monitoring that many people underestimate until they are living inside it.

This visibility changes how mistakes feel. Errors are not common—but uncertainty is. And uncertainty, when paired with visibility, can become emotionally expensive. You may find yourself replaying decisions, second-guessing language, or carrying responsibility for outcomes that were never fully within your control.

Then there is the toll of **expectation creep**.

The Nurse Practitioner role often expands quietly. What begins as scope flexibility can evolve into scope stretch. Additional patients. Additional coverage. Additional responsibilities justified by competence rather than capacity. The more capable you are, the more is often asked of you—without corresponding adjustments to time, support, or recovery.

None of this is inherently wrong. But it is cumulative.

The Toll Booth exists to slow you down before momentum takes over. Not to discourage you—but to clarify what you are agreeing to carry.

As you read the next section, you will see what the workday looks like when responsibility is no longer shared in the same way. Pay attention not just to tasks, but to *how the day feels.* Notice where your energy rises and where it drains.

The question is not whether you can pay the toll.

The question is whether you are willing to keep paying it—day after day—without losing the parts of yourself that matter outside of work.

Chapter 8
Introduction to the SCRUBfits™

Meet the SCRUB*fits*™

Every profession has its language.

In healthcare, that language usually sounds like credentials, specialties, and job titles. But anyone who has actually worked in this world knows something else is always happening underneath those labels. People cluster by rhythm, by tolerance for uncertainty, by how they carry responsibility, and by what drains them — or quietly brings them alive.

The **SCRUB*fits*™** exist to make that invisible layer visible.

They are not mascots. They are not stereotypes. They are not personality tests disguised as characters. The **SCRUB*fits*™** are alignment archetypes — narrative guides that represent the real ways people show up, survive, and thrive in healthcare work. Each **SCRUB*fits*™** voice reflects recognizable patterns: how someone thinks under pressure, how they relate to patients and teams, how they experience pace, autonomy, and responsibility, and how they sustain themselves over time. These guides are built from lived clinical reality, not theory alone.

In the Nurse Practitioner journey, one of the voices you will encounter is **Anna Remedy, DNP, FNP-BC, PMHNP**. Dr. Remedy does not appear to persuade you toward the profession or to simplify the demands it carries. Instead, she helps interpret what Nurse Practitioner work actually feels like — the cognitive load of decision-making, the quiet weight of accountability, the pace differences between practice settings, and the personal habits required to remain effective across a long career. Her reflections are designed to help you recognize not only what Nurse Practitioners do, but what the work asks of the person doing it.

You will encounter **SCRUB*fits*™** insights throughout the book — especially in the Day-in-the-Life chapters, career reflections, and key decision points where readers often pause and think: *Why does this part feel right to me — and that part doesn't?* The **SCRUB*fits*™** do not answer that question for you. They give you language to answer it yourself.

Think of them as mirrors, not models. You are not meant to become one. You are meant to recognize pieces of yourself across several. Some readers recognize themselves immediately. Others first notice contrast — *that is not me at all* — which is just as useful. There is no "best" **SCRUB*fits*™** and no hierarchy among them. There is only alignment, misalignment, and the clarity that comes from being able to name the difference.

Later in this book, you will encounter a short Mini **SCRUB*fits*™** Healthcare Career Assessment designed as a reflection tool rather than a test. For now, simply remember this: the **SCRUB*fits*™** exist to help you read these stories more clearly — and to remind you that if something does not fit, it does not mean you are wrong. It means the alignment deserves attention.

Chapter 9

Day in the Life Introduction

Introduction: 15 Days in the Life — Nurse Practitioner

The room is quiet except for the soft tick of a wall clock and the rustle of a paper gown. A patient sits on the edge of an exam table, eyes fixed on the floor. A knock, a gentle smile, a **stethoscope (gl)** catching the light.

In that narrow span between "Hi, I'm your Nurse Practitioner" and "Do you have any questions?" — that's where entire lives turn.

Spend A Day in the Life Across 15 Nurse Practitioner Specialties — Welcome into that space.

Think of this section as an invisible camera pass — not the glossy highlight reel, but the honest, behind-the-scenes cut. You'll slip into exam rooms just as the door closes, stand at ICU bedsides as alarms begin to crescendo, hover over NICU **isolettes (gl)** — glowing blue under **phototherapy lights (gl)**. You'll sit in on family conferences where no one quite knows what to ask, and you'll catch the small, almost-missed moments: the sigh of relief when a lab result finally comes back normal, the way a hand keeps reaching for a loved one's blanket long after that loved one has stepped out.

Over fifteen immersive days, you'll follow Nurse Practitioners across the full landscape of care:

- Community clinics where the waiting room hums in three languages at once.

- ICUs where seconds stretch long and the difference between "stable" and "crashing" is a drip titration.

- NICUs where entire shifts revolve around a baby gaining ten precious grams.

- Oncology suites where recliners, IV poles, and quiet courage share the same square footage.

- Behavioral health offices where the most important vital signs are the words people almost don't say out loud.

Each day drops you into a different vantage point: the Family NP building trust over flu shots and life advice; the Acute Care NP orchestrating a code in the ICU; the Neonatal NP counting breaths in heartbeats and grams; the Psychiatric NP holding space for stories that don't fit neatly into checkboxes. You'll watch them move through autonomy, ambiguity, and accountability — and feel the weight of what it means when your signature on an order set is also a promise to a family.

This isn't a protocol manual. It's a perspective map.

Because being an NP isn't just about writing the right orders — it's about reading the room, the body, and the story all at once. It's the discipline of:

- Seeing what others skim past
- Hearing what's buried under rehearsed answers
- Naming the thing nobody quite knows how to ask about

Every patient encounter is a set of data points — but also a confession. A negotiation. Sometimes a goodbye. Every shift demands not only clinical precision, but alignment — that inner "why" you lean on when the system is straining, the schedule is packed, and the easiest choice would be to stop caring so much.

You'll meet Nurse Practitioners who run on coffee, compassion, and the kind of dark humor that keeps teams functional at 03:00. They serve in:

- Disaster zones and delivery rooms
- School-based clinics and urban EDs
- Home health routes and cardiac ICUs
- Infusion chairs and psych intake rooms

You'll see them write orders with one hand while steadying a trembling shoulder with the other. You'll notice how leadership in this world rarely looks like a podium. More often, it looks like the person who knows when to speak up, when to sit down, and when to simply stay in the room.

Across these fifteen days, you'll watch a profession move fluidly between worlds: medicine and nursing, logic and empathy, urgency and stillness, leadership and lifelong learning. You'll see that for NPs, care doesn't end with the diagnosis; it extends into advocacy, education, follow-up calls on the drive home, and the quiet journaling they do before collapse, trying to make sense of all the small miracles and nearly-missed disasters.

15 Days in the Life — Nurse Practitioner is an invitation to see healthcare from the seat of both healer and human — to sit inside those conversations that usually happen after the door closes and the EMR (gl) — the electronic health record system where patient data is stored and managed — screen flickers to life.

Because the greatest medicine often begins not with a prescription, but with a sentence as simple — and as brave — as:

"Tell me what's been going on."

So step into the days — into the rounds, consults, triage calls, chart notes typed with cold coffee at the elbow, and the quiet exhale after a patient leaves. Listen for the heartbeat behind the stethoscope, the thought behind the pause, the conviction behind the signature.

Welcome to *15 Days in the Life — Nurse Practitioner* — a journey through care, clarity, and courage, told one patient, one choice, one heartbeat at a time.

Chapter 10

Day in the Life — Primary Care Nurse Practitioner

(Internal Medicine / Family Practice Clinic 08:00–17:30)

06:15 — Coffee, panels, and tiny boxes on a screen.

Ava sits at the kitchen table, hands wrapped around a mug that's finally hot enough to wake her up. Her laptop glows with the day's schedule in the clinic's EHR: sixteen "20-minute" slots that will never stay 20 minutes in real life.

She scrolls down the list:

Annual wellness visit, 72-year-old with "fatigue."

Chronic disease follow-up: diabetes, hypertension, chronic kidney disease (CKD).

Same-day "sore throat, rule-out strep."

Follow-up for anxiety and insomnia.

"Medication check" for a long list of prescriptions that never quite come in a tidy bag.

A late afternoon “new patient: multiple issues.” The phrase makes her smile ruefully. Everyone is a multiple issue; the system is the one that gets 20 minutes.

Her wife, Lena, shuffles in, hair in a loose bun, reaching for the coffee pot. “You look like you’re already on visit number six,” she says.

“Just previewing today’s roller coaster,” Ava answers. “I think the theme is going to be ‘Everything hurts and my lab portal is scary.’”

Lena kisses her cheek. “You’re good at un-scaring things,” she says. “Just remember that someone might walk out feeling better about their entire life because of a sentence you think is obvious.”

Ava closes the laptop, tucks that reminder into her mental pocket, and goes to get ready.

07:30 — Drive, dashboards, and mental math.

On the drive to the clinic, the sky is turning from gray to pale blue. Ava puts on music she barely hears, her brain already sorting through clinical checklists.

Her panel management dashboard has been nagging her all week:

Diabetes patients overdue for A1C.

Those missing colon cancer screening (colonoscopy or stool tests).

Women due for cervical cancer screening (Pap test).

Patients over 65 without an advance directive on file.

She thinks about Mr. Rodriguez, whose blood pressure has been creeping up, and Ms. Hill, who swore she would schedule her mammogram "next month" six months ago. Primary care is less about dramatic saves and more about a thousand tiny course corrections that prevent disasters no one will ever see.

The clinic building appears ahead: a low brick structure between a grocery store and a bus stop. Most of her patients live within a few miles, but their lives span a much wider range than the map suggests.

07:50 — Pre-clinic: inbox triage before the first hello.

In the cramped provider workroom, Ava logs into the EHR and opens her inbox. It's already full.

Refill requests: "Out of my blood pressure meds—pharmacy says they faxed twice."

Portal messages: "My sugar has been high all week, what do I do?" "Can you explain my lab results?"

Test results: an A1C back at 9.8%, a PSA mildly elevated, a low eGFR (glomerular filtration rate) (gl) that means someone's kidneys are not as happy as they look on the outside.

She responds quickly where she can:

Refills approved with a note: "Please keep your appointment on Thursday so we can talk about how things are going."

Reassurance plus action steps: "Your cholesterol looks better; let's keep the statin going. Your A1C is higher—we'll talk at your visit today."

A few results she flags: "This needs a phone call, not a portal note." Bad news should not arrive like a package on a doorstep.

By the time the medical assistant sticks her head in—"Your eight o'clock is here"—Ava has made a small dent in the invisible part of her job that never appears on the schedule.

08:00 — Annual wellness: fatigue, "just getting older," and hidden depression.

Mrs. Ellis, 72, sits on the exam table, small frame swallowed in a floral blouse. She's here for her Medicare wellness visit, but when Ava asks, "What brought you in today?" she answers, "I'm just tired all the time."

The templates offer checkboxes: fall risk, cognitive screen, depression screening (PHQ-9) (gl), vaccination status. Ava uses them, but she doesn't let them use her.

They talk through the basics: sleep, appetite, pain, bowel habits, medication list. The med list alone takes several minutes—blood pressure pills, a statin, something for reflux, a sleeping pill she's been on "for years," two herbal supplements a friend recommended.

At first, Mrs. Ellis chalks everything up to "getting older," but when Ava asks the PHQ-9 questions gently, she sees the pattern.

"More days than not, I just don't see the point of getting dressed," Mrs. Ellis admits quietly. "I do it anyway, but it feels like I'm walking through mud."

Ava leans in slightly. "Have you had any thoughts that you'd be better off not here?" she asks.

"Not like... doing anything to myself," Mrs. Ellis says. "Just... If I didn't wake up one morning, it wouldn't be the worst thing."

Together, they work through possibilities: medical causes (anemia, thyroid issues, sleep apnea) and the very real possibility of depression layered on top of loneliness after her husband's death. Ava orders labs, refers her to a grief-support group, discusses starting a low-dose antidepressant, and screens for safety.

Before she leaves, Ava asks, "What's one small thing you used to enjoy that we could try to make room for again?"

Mrs. Ellis thinks for a moment. "I used to like sitting in the park watching the ducks," she says.

"Then that's our homework," Ava replies. "One duck-sitting session in the next week. Health includes ducks."

09:00 — Diabetes, numbers, and negotiating real life.

Next is Mr. Khan, 58, whose A1C came back at 9.8%. He settles into the chair, arms crossed. "I knew it would be bad," he says. "Just tell me how much I've failed."

Ava swivels the monitor so they can look together. "This number is a piece of information," she says. "Not a moral grade. It's telling us your blood sugar has been higher than we want, which means higher risk for problems with your eyes, kidneys, nerves, and heart. But it's also telling us where we can make changes."

They review his current regimen: metformin twice a day, a sulfonylurea (gl) he sometimes forgets, lifestyle plans that never quite stick because he works nights at a warehouse and grabs whatever is available in the vending machines.

She asks specific questions about his days instead of lecturing about carbs in the abstract. "What does a usual meal look like at 2 a.m. on your shift? What's actually available?"

He laughs, a little bitter. "Chips, candy bars, maybe a sad sandwich."

They brainstorm realistic swaps and small changes instead of imaginary perfect meals. Then they discuss adding a GLP-1 receptor agonist (gl) injection, explaining how it works, side effects, and—crucially—the cost.

"That's the problem," he says. "Last time someone gave me a new med, I got to the pharmacy and they wanted $300."

Ava nods. "I never want you to be surprised at the counter," she says. "Let me have our pharmacist check your insurance coverage and see if there's a patient assistance program (gl). If this ends up too expensive, we'll adjust the plan."

They set a specific, achievable goal: walking 15 minutes on his days off, checking his blood sugar twice a day, bringing his glucometer next visit.

As he leaves, his shoulders are a little less slumped. "Thanks for not just telling me to 'eat better,'" he says. "I've heard that for twenty years."

"Specific problems, specific plans," Ava replies. "That's our deal."

10:00 — Sick visit: sore throat, strip tests, and health anxiety.

The next patient, a college student named Mariah, sits on the exam table scrolling her phone, mask slightly askew. “I think I have strep,” she says before Ava even sits down. “My roommate had it last week.”

A quick history reveals a sore throat for two days, mild fever, some runny nose. No cough, no trouble breathing, no difficulty swallowing.

Ava examines her throat, palpates tender lymph nodes, and explains the Centor criteria (gl) in simple terms. “Based on your symptoms, it’s reasonable to do a rapid strep test. If it’s positive, antibiotics. If not, we treat it like a viral infection and focus on comfort.”

The test is negative. Mariah looks crestfallen and oddly anxious. “But I feel awful,” she says. “Are you sure it’s not something serious?”

Ava recognizes the familiar mix of physical discomfort and health anxiety fueled by late-night internet searches. She validates her misery without feeding the panic.

“You feel bad, and that is real,” she says. “It’s just that the cause looks like a virus, and antibiotics don’t help viruses. They only give you side effects and contribute to antibiotic resistance.”

She prints clear instructions, including red-flag symptoms. Before Mariah leaves, she adds, “Just because it’s ‘only’ viral doesn’t mean you have to tough it out alone. If you’re not improving in a few days, let us know.”

Sometimes, the most important prescription is a roadmap.

11:00 — Multi-problem visit: the 20-minute impossible.

A 40-year-old new patient, Mr. Thompson, is booked as a "new patient, multiple issues." On his intake form he's checked off: back pain, headaches, "stomach issues," and "trouble sleeping." He also circled "stress: high" three times.

"I know I'm not supposed to bring a list," he says, pulling out a folded sheet of paper anyway. "But I brought a list."

Ava smiles. "Lists are welcome," she says. "Our job is to figure out what we can realistically tackle today and what we need to schedule follow-ups for."

They triage together. Back pain for five years, worse after long days at his warehouse job. Headaches that sound like tension headaches, sometimes migraines. Stomach issues linked to fast food, irregular meals, and maybe stress more than anything sinister. Sleep disrupted by pain and worry.

There is no way to fix five years of accumulated problems in one visit, and she refuses to pretend otherwise.

"Here's what I propose," she says. "Today we focus on your back pain and sleep, because those affect everything else. We'll do a basic exam, maybe some labs to rule out anything serious, start treatment there. Then we book follow-up visits specifically for headaches and stomach issues."

They agree on stretching and strengthening exercises, a referral to physical therapy, a short course of anti-inflammatory medication, and basic sleep hygiene changes. She screens for depression and anxiety; both show up. They talk about therapy options and, if needed, a future visit to discuss medications.

He relaxes a little as the plan takes shape. "I thought you were going to tell me I'm a mess," he says.

"You are a person whose life is heavy," Ava replies. "Our job is to pick up one corner of the load at a time, not pretend we can lift the whole thing in one go."

12:30 — Lunch, lab results, and the phone calls no one sees.

Officially, it's lunch. In reality, Ava heats her food and eats it at her desk while calling patients whose results deserve a voice.

She phones a man whose PSA is elevated. "This doesn't mean you have prostate cancer," she explains. "It means we need to look closer. I'd like you to see urology."

She calls a woman whose mammogram picked up a suspicious lesion. Ava avoids vague phrases like "abnormal" and gives concrete next steps: diagnostic imaging, referral to breast surgery clinic. She pauses often to let the questions and fear surface.

She reviews a slightly low kidney function on a patient taking multiple blood pressure and pain meds. She adjusts doses, orders repeat labs, sends a portal message summarizing the changes in plain language.

By the time her 13:00 patient has been roomed, her lunch is half-eaten, but five people know what's happening in their bodies and what the plan is. That counts.

13:00 — Telehealth: screens, connection, and meeting people where they are.

The next appointment is virtual. Ms. Rivera appears on the screen, sitting in her car between cleaning jobs. Children's backpacks are visible in the back seat.

"I'm sorry," she says breathlessly. "I couldn't take off work, but I didn't want to miss this."

They're following up on hypertension and depression. Ava reviews her home blood pressure readings, which are better since titrating her medication and shifting her schedule to include a brief daily walk.

"How's your mood?" Ava asks.

"Still up and down," Ms. Rivera says. "But the downs don't feel as deep. I started journaling like you said. And I actually went to that support group at the community center."

They adjust her antidepressant dose slightly and make a concrete plan for the next month that fits into her reality: quick microwaveable meals that aren't all instant noodles, five-minute breathing exercises between houses, enlisting her teenage daughter to help remind her about meds.

A toddler suddenly appears in the back seat, waving at the camera.

"This is Sofia," Ms. Rivera says, laughing. "She wanted to say hi."

Ava waves back. "Hi, Sofia. Your mom is doing really hard work," she says.

When the call ends, Ava marvels again at how medicine has shifted: half clinic, half wherever people can find a quiet-ish corner and a reasonably stable connection.

14:30 — Vaccines, prevention, and the long game.

Back in the exam room, Ava sees a middle-aged man for a "routine check-up." He insists he's "never sick" and only came because his partner threatened to drag him in.

On review, he hasn't seen a clinician in eight years. He has no idea what his blood pressure runs, eats fast food most days, and has a family history of colon cancer and early heart disease.

"Feeling fine is wonderful," Ava says. "My job is to keep it that way as long as we can."

They talk screening: colon cancer (colonoscopy vs stool tests), blood pressure, cholesterol, diabetes. She recommends vaccines he's due for: tetanus booster, shingles vaccine, an updated COVID and flu shot. He makes a face at the idea of multiple injections.

"Think of it this way," she says. "Would you rather have one sore arm this week, or be in the ICU with something we could have prevented? I'm pro-sore-arm."

He laughs and, in the end, rolls up his sleeve. They order labs, schedule a follow-up, and talk about one small change he's willing to make for his heart: swapping soda for water at least half the time.

Primary care's victories are often invisible—diseases that never happen. She's okay with that.

16:00 — Late-day curveball: chest pain in a 15-minute slot.

Her 16:00 appointment is booked as "follow-up for reflux," but as soon as Mr. Patel sits down, Ava knows this isn't going to be a quick visit.

"My chest has been hurting more," he says. "I thought it was heartburn, but yesterday it went into my arm."

The hairs on the back of her neck stand up. She takes a rapid-focused history: onset, character, radiation, associated symptoms. She checks his vitals, listens to his heart and lungs, notes the risk factors she already knows from his chart: high blood pressure, high cholesterol, family history of early heart disease.

"Right now, I can't safely call this 'just reflux,'" she says. "I want you evaluated in the emergency department to rule out a heart attack (myocardial infarction) (gl)."

He hesitates. "Do I have to? I don't want to overreact."

Ava meets his eyes. "You are not overreacting," she says firmly. "If this is your heart, time matters. If it's not, we'll both be relieved. But we won't know unless they evaluate you there."

She calls report to the ED, arranges transport, prints a summary of his history. Later, she'll check his chart from home to see what they found, even though it's technically after hours. Once you send someone down that hallway, you don't stop caring at the clinic door.

17:15 — The inbox avalanche and unfinished lists.

Official clinic hours end at 17:00, but Ava's computer screen still glows. She finishes a few last notes, sends referrals, and answers the most urgent remaining messages:

"Yes, your imaging was normal—your pain is real even if the scan doesn't show a cause. Let's talk next week about managing it."

"Your thyroid level is off; I've adjusted your dose. Here's how to take the new pill."

"Please schedule a follow-up so we can discuss your sleep and anxiety in more detail."

She leaves some non-urgent messages for tomorrow. Primary care has taught her that there will always be more to do, and that the work is a relay, not a sprint she can win alone.

Before she logs out, she opens the panel dashboard again and clicks a reminder for herself about the patients overdue for screening. The list is long. So is her commitment.

18:10 — Home, leftovers, and redefining "saving lives."

At home, Lena has leftover stir-fry warmed on the stove and the dog sprawled in the middle of the kitchen like a hazard that wags.

"How many lives did you save today?" Lena teases, the question they've joked about since Ava left hospital nursing for clinic life.

"Hard to say," Ava answers, setting her bag down. "Maybe one in the ED, maybe a few hearts and kidneys ten years from now, maybe one soul that decided to stay. Mostly I adjusted meds, explained lab results, begged people to stop smoking, and tried to make scary things less scary."

"Sounds like saving lives, just on a different timeline," Lena says.

Later, on the couch, Ava opens her journal.

She writes:

"Primary care is where the big, messy stories start and where they come back when the hospital is done. It's where prevention sneaks in between refills and sore throats, where we trade in small conversations that add up to fewer strokes, fewer amputations, fewer lonely hearts. No one claps when a heart attack never happens, but that doesn't mean it wasn't prevented."

She closes the notebook, turns off the lamp, and leans into the quiet. Tomorrow, the schedule squares will fill up again with new names and old ones.

Same work: standing at the front door of the health system, listening deeply, and helping people carry their lives one visit at a time.

SCRUB*fits*™ Reflection — Anna Remedy, DNP, FNP-BC

"Primary care Nurse Practitioner work often looks steady from the outside, but inside each visit is a rapid series of decisions balancing prevention, chronic disease management, and patient education. Some clinicians thrive in this continuity-driven environment where long-term relationships guide clinical judgment. Others find the constant balancing of time pressure and complex patient needs exhausting. Pay attention to how this pace feels to you. Alignment in primary care is not about how busy the schedule is — it is about whether relationship-based care energizes you over the long term."

Chapter 11

Day in the Life — Acute Care Nurse Practitioner

(Hospital ICU · 07:00–19:00)

04:45 — Lo-fi jazz and worst-case scenarios

The alarm hums softly, then swells into lo-fi beats. Darius blinks awake, staring at the ceiling while his brain boots up ahead of his body: ventilator settings, vasopressor drips (gl), septic shock, yesterday's post-arrest whose lactate (gl) refused to cooperate. Worst-case scenarios queue up before his feet hit the floor.

Beside him, Naomi is a warm shape under the covers.

"ICU day?" she murmurs.

"Yeah."

She reaches for his wrist. "Be safe."

He leans down, kisses her forehead. "Be smart."

Their ritual holds. She smiles without fully waking.

05:00 — Breakfast and headcount

In the kitchen, the local news murmurs while Darius flips eggs over avocado toast, slices a banana, and pours black coffee strong enough to power a code cart.

Juniper, their tabby cat, weaves between his ankles, tail flicking.

"You're the only one who doesn't page me," he tells her.

He eats standing at the counter, scrolling through the ICU census on his phone: septic shock, ARDS (gl), post-CABG (gl), post-arrest hypothermia (gl). Names steady him. The known is easier than the unknown.

05:30 — Driving into someone else's worst day

The city is half-asleep — streetlights still glowing, sky smudged pink at the horizon. Darius drives with his coffee thermos in the cupholder, lo-fi still playing low.

He runs mental checklists: delirium screening, sedation holidays, vent weaning, antibiotic coverage. Wonders if Bed 12's MAP (gl) held. Hopes the family in Bed 14 actually went home to sleep.

The hospital rises ahead, glass reflecting the early light. The building never sleeps. Neither do the problems inside it.

06:40 — The ICU hum

The unit doors swish open. Cool, dry air. The hiss of ventilators. Overlapping monitor tones in different rhythms. Coffee, chlorhexidine (gl), and something metallic beneath it all.

"Morning, D," a night RN calls from the desk.

"How bad?"

"Four fresh admits and one still on pressors. We saved the fun ones for you."

He scans the whiteboard — bed numbers compressed into diagnoses. He slings his stethoscope around his neck and shifts from human tired to clinical sharp.

07:00 — Handoff: passing the night into the day

The team clusters: night NP, day NP, bedside nurses, charge, residents.

"Bed 12 — septic, cultures pending, norepinephrine (gl) at 0.12, lactate trending down."

"Bed 14 — STEMI (gl) post-CABG (gl), intubated, EF rough."

"Bed 15 — neuro trauma, ICP (gl) stable."

"Bed 16 — vent weaned overnight, possible extubation."

Darius scribbles shorthand only he understands. By the end, he knows the unit's weather — no active storm, but a thin margin before one.

07:30 — Rounds: orchestra in scrubs

They move room to room: attending, Darius, residents, bedside nurses, pharmacist, dietitian, RT.

Ventilators hiss like second heartbeats. Decisions stack quickly. Pressors are adjusted. Sedation is debated. Spontaneous breathing trials (gl) planned. Nothing is theoretical anymore.

08:30 — Chasing pressure, catching details

Bed 12's MAP drifts again. The arterial line (gl) waveform looks dampened. Darius recalibrates the transducer (gl), orders a fluid bolus, repeats the lactate.

"Think of it as topping off the tank," he tells the nurse.

He rests a hand on the bed rail, speaking anyway.

"We're still with you."

Small adjustments. Big stakes.

10:30 — Code Blue: time goes sideways

"Code Blue, Bed 10."

Conversation drops mid-word. Darius is already moving. Compressions. Epinephrine. Rhythm checks. The defibrillator (gl) whines. Shock delivered. Time collapses to muscle memory and commands.

"ROSC (gl)!"

A fragile rhythm returns. Sweat cools on his neck. The nurse meets his eyes; they exchange a brief nod. They got this one back.

There is no pause to process it. The unit keeps moving.

11:45 — ICU lunch

Yogurt, granola, and an energy drink at the nurses' station. He dictates notes into Epic, adjusts heparin (gl), answers resident questions between bites.

At the far end of the hall, a family hovers at a doorway. Darius notices. He always notices.

12:30 — Family meeting: choosing each word like glass

The conference room is quiet. A box of tissues sits untouched. A woman and her teenage son sit across from Darius and the attending.

“We’ve thrown everything we can at this,” Darius says carefully, imaging and lab trends spread out. “His lungs, his heart, his kidneys — they’re all struggling.”

“So what does that mean?” she asks.

“It means we’re at a crossroads,” he says. “We can keep going, knowing it’s unlikely to change the outcome. Or we can shift our focus to comfort — to honoring what he would have wanted.”

He lets the silence stretch.

“We’ll stay with you,” he adds softly. “All of it.”

Tears fall. Nobody looks at the clock. This is Nurse Practitioner work as much as any medication order.

19:30 — After the monitors go quiet

Sign-out complete, Darius leaves with shoulders heavy and thoughts still buzzing. The drive home is silent. Music off. City lights blur past.

At home, Juniper greets him like nothing else exists. Naomi listens as he recounts the day in fragments. He showers. The water runs hot. The adrenaline finally drains.

Later, lying in the dark, the question surfaces — not dramatically, just honestly:

Could I do this again tomorrow?

He doesn't answer it tonight.

SCRUB*fits*™ Reflection — Anna Remedy, DNP, FNP-BC

"Acute care Nurse Practitioner roles demand comfort with urgency, rapid assessment, and high-stakes decision-making. For clinicians who naturally think quickly under pressure, these environments can feel engaging and purposeful. For others, the same intensity can create long-term strain even when performance is strong. The key question is not whether you can function in high-acuity settings, but whether that sustained level of urgency feels sustainable across years of practice."

Chapter 12

Day in the Life — Palliative Care Nurse Practitioner

(Hospital Consult Service & Home Hospice Visits 08:00–18:00)

06:00 — Tea, sunrise, and the weight of words

Talia wakes before her alarm, as she often does. Outside the bedroom window, the city is still gray and undecided about the day. Inside, the house hums quietly with heat and appliances.

She makes chamomile tea with honey and sits at the kitchen table with her planner. Today's list looks different than most: two hospital palliative-care consults, three home hospice visits, and a family meeting flagged as "likely goals of care shift."

She taps her pen, thinking less about medications than language — the sentences that might change the shape of someone's life. In palliative care, words matter as much as morphine.

06:45 — Scrubs, sweater, and a soft armor

Soft navy scrubs, a long cardigan — professional but human. She packs her bag: stethoscope, tablet with Epic (gl), POLST (Physician Orders for Life-Sustaining Treatment) (gl) forms, advance directive (gl) information, a small book of poems, travel-size tissues.

Her partner, Eli, meets her at the door. “Text me if you need to breathe.”

Sometimes she does. Sometimes she doesn’t realize she needed to until later.

07:30 — Hospital corridors and consult lists

The hospital is already awake — transporters, nurses, residents clutching coffee. In the consult office, the team reviews the day: metastatic pancreatic cancer on Oncology, ARDS (acute respiratory distress syndrome) (gl) on ECMO (extracorporeal membrane oxygenation) (gl) in the MICU, end-stage heart failure with repeated admissions.

Talia takes Oncology and MICU this morning. She logs into Epic. The numbers tell one story. The people will tell another.

08:15 — Oncology consult: pain and the truth under “I’m fine”

Room 512 smells faintly of floral lotion and antiseptic. Mr. Harris lies in bed, IV pump ticking. His daughter sits nearby, laptop closed.

“I’m fine,” he says.

Talia pulls up a chair. “On a scale of zero to ten, how ‘fine’ is your pain?”

"Seven," he admits.

They talk specifics — burning versus aching, baseline pain versus spikes. She adjusts his regimen: a slight increase in long-acting opioid (gl), better breakthrough dosing (gl), low-dose dexamethasone (gl), a different antiemetic (gl).

Then she shifts. "What have you understood about what's happening with your cancer?"

He looks away. His daughter's hands still. They talk about what matters, about documenting wishes so decisions don't fall entirely on his daughter's shoulders. When Talia leaves, his pain has eased — and the unspoken has finally been named.

10:00 — MICU consult: machines, numbers, and meaning

Room 210 is dim, alive with wires and soft mechanical sounds. A woman in her 30s lies sedated, ventilator and ECMO circuit doing most of the work. The team worries support is prolonging suffering.

In the family room, Talia sits rather than stands. She explains the situation plainly. "We're at a crossroads. We can continue as we are, knowing the outcome may not change, or we can shift our focus to comfort."

They talk about who their daughter is — independent, adventurous, never wanting to live on machines indefinitely. No decisions today, just the beginning of letting go.

12:30 — Cafeteria food and emotional triage

Soup grows cold as Talia meets with the social worker and chaplain. They compare notes — families in distress, staff near breaking. The pager vibrates before she finishes eating.

13:30 — Home hospice: dog hair, oxygen tubing, and ordinary grace

The afternoon brings home visits. Mr. Jenkins, 87, sits in a recliner, oxygen cannula (gl) in place, dog hair clinging to his slippers.

She listens, adjusts opioid dosing for dyspnea (gl), and deprescribes medications meant for years he won't have. Statins. Vitamins. A bisphosphonate (gl).

"Fewer pills, more pie," he jokes.

His daughter hovers. Talia reminds her: hospice is there so she can be a daughter, not a nurse.

15:00 — Hospice bed: music, morphine, and last wishes

Ms. Alvarez lies in a hospice bed beneath family photos, a Spanish ballad playing softly. Pain is three, maybe four. Talia adjusts morphine, confirms DNR/DNI (do not resuscitate, do not intubate) (gl), reinforces her wish to stay home.

"You're doing a beautiful job," she tells the son holding his mother's hand.

16:30 — The drive between worlds

Talia sits in her car for a moment before driving on. ICU machines in the morning, oxygen concentrators (gl) and casseroles in the afternoon. Different worlds, same work.

17:15 — Back to MICU: decisions and the grace of "enough"

The family has decided. Comfort-focused care. Talia explains what withdrawal of ECMO and the ventilator will look like, answers hard questions without flinching.

When the machines are turned off, the room fills with quiet grief instead of alarms. Afterward, a nurse whispers, "It feels like I failed."

"You didn't," Talia says. "You carried her as far as medicine could. Then you helped her leave gently."

18:30 — Notes, night, and one line

Late at home, Talia finishes notes in Epic. The chart is careful and clinical. The day was not.

In her journal, she writes:

"Palliative care is not giving up. It is telling the truth when cures are gone and staying anyway. Morphine, paperwork, and hand-holding all count as medicine."

Tomorrow will bring more consults, more homes, more goodbyes.

Same work — walking with people at the edge and reminding them they are not alone there.

Chapter 13

Day in the Life — Family Nurse Practitioner, Rural

(Community Health Clinic · 08:00–16:30)

06:00 — The coffee pot and the first chart of the day

The coffee pot gurgles before dawn, sputtering like it's not sure it's ready either. Tanya's kitchen glows amber, the only light on in the house. She sits at the table in navy scrubs, tablet propped against a cereal box, scrolling through today's schedule in Epic — coughs, chronic disease follow-ups, an "establish care" that could be anything, and a walk-in already flagged as "complex."

Behind her, Miguel measures oats into a pot while their twins, Maya and Leo, argue over the blue bowl. Baxter, their rescued beagle mix, patrols the floor. A strawberry drops. Baxter pounces.

"That's fruit privilege," Tanya murmurs, eyes still on the tablet.

Breakfast becomes a fast montage — spoons clinking, backpacks zipping, someone yelling "Where are my shoes?"

She answers a portal message about a lisinopril refill between sips of coffee. This is the pre-shift: ordinary life before she steps into everyone else's.

06:45 — Lunch packed, armor on

She snaps the lid on her chickpea salad, adds a banana and trail mix, and pours coffee strong enough to chart its own vitals. The twins press against the front window, palms flat, Baxter wedged between them.

"Love you!"

"Love you more!"

Driving away, patient names already scroll through her head: reorder albuterol, check that elevated A1C, remember Mrs. Greene's granddaughter's name. By the time she hits the main road, Tanya is no longer just a mom leaving home. She's the NP people will call their provider today.

07:25 — Commute as calibration

Same route. Same podcast — today on rural health disparities. Care shouldn't depend on your ZIP code, the host says. Tanya looks out at the fields: not quite rural, not quite suburban, definitely under-resourced.

The community clinic sits one block from the grocery store, one from the church, near the bus stop where kids gather after school. Half gravel parking lot, half cracked asphalt. To Tanya, it might as well be marble. This is where people come when they have nowhere else to go.

07:55 — Walking into the day

Fluorescent lights too bright for the hour. The front desk is already busy. Someone's kid is sick. Someone missed their ride. Someone wants to "just ask the nurse a quick question."

"Morning, Ms. G."

"Morning, FNP Tanya! Flu clinic overflow — we're swimming in sniffles."

"Good," Tanya grins. "Let's make immunity fashionable."

She logs into Epic. The schedule fills the screen like a Tetris board with no pause button.

08:00 — Room 2: a farmer, a knee, and a deadline

Calloused hands, oil-stained nails — the kind that don't come in unless something's wrong.

"Knee again?"

"I'm fine."

The wince says otherwise. Tanya palpates the joint, explains early osteoarthritis, orders an X-ray, adjusts his NSAID (gl) plan, sets a follow-up reminder.

"We caught it early," she says. "Let's manage it now so it doesn't manage you later."

One room down. Fourteen to go.

08:45 — Room 4: tiny lungs, big worry

The toddler's cough rattles. Tanya warms her Littmann before listening — faint wheeze, tight airways.

"Good news," she tells the mother. "I know what to do."

Nebulizer (gl). Spacer (gl). A Paw Patrol sticker stuck to her scrub top. While mist curls around the child's face, Tanya explains asthma triggers and inhaler technique in plain language. Afterward, the wheeze softens. Breathing finds room again.

09:30 — Room 1: one negative test, ten unasked questions

The pregnancy test is negative. Relief and disappointment flicker together.

"So," Tanya says gently, "what do you want long-term?"

They talk contraception, partners who don't listen, a future the patient hasn't felt allowed to design.

"You deserve care before crisis," Tanya says.

The patient leaves with a plan — and agency.

10:45 — Room 5: numbers, nuance, and a glucometer

Type 2 diabetes. Three months in. The glucometer (gl) log is imperfect but trending down.

"See this?" Tanya points. "That matters."

They adjust metformin, talk honestly about soda and late-night snacks, set one achievable goal. In Epic, the note will read: A1C improving; regimen adjusted.

What it won't show: posture shifting from defeated to maybe.

SCRUB*fits*™ Reflection — Anna Remedy, DNP, FNP-BC, PMHNP

"Rural Nurse Practitioner practice often expands both autonomy and responsibility. Resources may be limited, referral networks farther away, and clinical independence greater than many new graduates expect. Some clinicians find this autonomy deeply rewarding, while others prefer the support structure of larger systems. Notice whether the independence described in this chapter feels empowering or isolating. That reaction can be one of the clearest signals of long-term alignment."

Chapter 14

Day in the Life — Pediatric Nurse Practitioner

(Children's Primary Care Clinic · 07:30–15:30)

05:45 — Alarm, tiny feet, and pancake negotiations

The alarm hums, but the real wake-up is the thump of small feet racing down the hall. Before Sam fully opens her eyes, six-year-old twins Eli and Nora cannonball onto the bed, dinosaur blankets tangled around them.

"Mommy, pancakes?" Nora mumbles.

"Mini pancakes," Sam says. "Clinic day, not Sunday brunch."

From the kitchen, Jordan calls, "Too late — I promised heart-shaped ones!"

Maple, their golden doodle, bounds up next, tail wagging dangerously fast. Sam's first assessment of the day: two hyper, one hungry, one fluffy — all stable.

06:00 — Pancake clinic

Coffee and batter fill the kitchen. Jordan flips heart-shaped banana pancakes while the twins argue about dragons versus astronauts. Sam cradles her mug like an IV infusion and scrolls through the clinic EHR — eight well-child checks, two asthma follow-ups, a behavior consult flagged yellow, and flu shots. So many flu shots.

She recognizes names instantly — the toddler who fears stethoscopes, the nine-year-old who wants to be a cardiologist, the teenager whose answer to everything is "fine."

"Power up," Jordan says, sliding her a plate.

"Your faith in stickers is inspiring," Sam replies.

Lunches get packed. A permission slip appears out of nowhere. The usual chaos.

06:40 — Stars, pockets, and armor

Sam pulls on navy scrubs dotted with silver stars — clinic-approved and kid-enticing. She loads her pockets: penlight (gl), pens, alcohol pads, growth-chart reference, YOU DID IT! stickers.

She helps Eli find a missing shoe, reminds Nora not to eat floor snacks, and kisses Jordan goodbye.

"Good luck with flu shot day, warrior," Jordan says.

"Good luck with gravity," Sam replies — Jordan's a pediatric physical therapist.

06:55 — Carpool karaoke and invisible prep

The twins belt out a song about a dancing avocado on the drive to school. At drop-off, Sam crouches.

“You got this,” she tells Eli.

“No eating art supplies,” she tells Nora.

“Can I tell my teacher you give shots?” Nora asks.

“Tell her I give bravery superpowers.”

She watches them disappear into backpacks, then turns toward the clinic. Her brain switches from spelling words to vaccine schedules without hesitation.

07:20 — Murals, mist, and morning huddle

The clinic’s murals glow in the morning mist — giraffes, rockets, sea creatures. Inside, cartoon voices mix with the soundtrack of early-morning meltdowns.

Huddle is fast: vaccine stock good, grape flavoring gone, behavior consult at 10:15, and “the biter” returning at 11.

“Guess I’ll wear my bite-resistant armor,” Sam says.

She checks her otoscope (gl), tongue depressors, and calibrates the pediatric scale (gl) — the yellow one with duck stickers that somehow makes toddlers braver.

08:00 — Two-month well baby: squeaks and stats

Hazel, two months old, arrives bundled like a floral burrito. Her parents hover, exhausted and anxious.

“She makes this squeak,” Dad says.

Sam listens — heart rapid and steady, lungs clear, reflexes

perfect. She walks them through growth percentiles, safe sleep, tummy time, and realistic expectations about sleep.

"Those squeaks?" Sam says. "Totally normal newborn opera."

Vaccines come next. Hazel's cry slices through the hallway, then fades to hiccups.

"You just bought her superpowers," Sam says. "No guilt required."

08:45 — Asthma check: superhero training

Marcus, nine, flashes LED sneakers and proudly presents his peak flows. They review his asthma action plan (gl), inhaler technique with a spacer (gl), and symptom patterns.

"You're officially a respiratory pro," Sam says, adjusting his inhaled corticosteroid (gl) dose. "Teach the residents."

She prints a new school plan and adds, "Text if you score a goal. Both are important."

09:30 — Earache, lion, and bubblegum meds

Four-year-old DeShawn stomps in clutching a stuffed lion.

"My ear is mad."

Sam peers in: red, bulging tympanic membrane (gl). Acute otitis media (gl). She explains amoxicillin (gl), pain control, and warning signs.

To DeShawn: "Bubblegum medicine that fights ear germs."

Lion gets a sticker. DeShawn gets two.

10:15 — Behavior consult: worry in a small hoodie

Eleven-year-old Maya perches on the exam table, hoodie pulled tight. School has been hard. Sleep is worse.

Sam closes the laptop and listens. They name anxiety disorders (gl) without labels that scare, build language around "false fire alarms," and outline a plan — counseling, coping tools, follow-up.

"You're not broken," Sam says. "Your brain's just loud."

Maya nods. The room feels lighter.

11:30 — Catch-up: snacks, notes, and vaccine math

Sam eats standing up while finishing notes and triple-checking vaccine fridge (gl) temperatures. Her documentation is clean and clinical. The emotional labor stays invisible.

Then the MA appears. "The biter's here."

Sam exhales. "Send stickers. And backup."

12:00 — Biter, immunity, and tactical distraction

Three-year-old Liam glares from inside a dinosaur hoodie. Sam deploys distraction: toy otoscope, bubbles, a story about dinosaurs who get superhero juice.

Two pokes. One scream. One attempted bite diverted into foam.

"Vaccines given; tolerated with expected distress," she documents.

Translation: nobody bled.

13:15 — Lunch-that-isn't, part two

Half a sandwich, clinic gossip, and a portal photo of a lacy rash. Fifth disease (gl). Sam replies with reassurance and red flags, then finishes the sandwich anyway.

14:00 — Sports physical and invisible screening

Jaden wants clearance for basketball. Sam checks vitals, vision screening (gl), heart, lungs, joints — then asks the questions that aren't on the form.

"How's your sleep?"

"How's your mood?"

They talk pressure and the myth that toughness means silence.

On the form: CLEARED.

In the note: stress discussed; monitor.

15:10 — Last visits, last stickers, last messages

The afternoon blurs: constipation confessions, eczema flares, flat-foot reassurance. ADHD refills, school forms, vaccine lot numbers.

One portal message reads, "Is it normal to feel like I'm failing?"

Sam types back: "Feeling like you're failing usually means you care deeply."

15:40 — Exit through the mural jungle

She logs out of the EHR, hangs up her stethoscope, and walks past yawning toddlers clutching sticker sheets. The murals glow in afternoon light.

Today, she shepherded a small universe through growing up.

16:10 — Home: tacos, homework, and decompression

The twins tackle her at the door.

"Did you give shots?"

"Yes."

"Did anyone cry?"

"Yes."

"They were brave anyway," she adds.

Dinner smells like tacos. Nobody needs vitals. Nobody needs a weight percentile.

20:30 — Storytime and reflection

Later, journal open, Sam lists the day's small bravery: Hazel's squeaks, Marcus's pride, Maya's quiet fear, Liam's almost-bite.

She writes:

"Pediatrics is tiny courage on repeat. My job isn't just catching illness. It's catching the moment someone says, 'I'm scared,' and answering, 'I've got you.'"

She turns off the light, listening to her own kids sleep.

Tomorrow: more stickers, more tears, more giggles.

Same mission — keeping small bodies and big feelings safe in a loud world.

Chapter 15

Day in the Life — Reproductive Health Nurse Practitioner

(OB/GYN & Reproductive Health Clinic · 08:00–16:30)

05:30 — Moonlight, messages, and mental triage.

Lena's alarm hums while the moon still clings to the sky. She gives herself one quiet minute before the day begins — before contraception decisions, abnormal Pap results, bleeding that isn't normal, and questions that don't fit neatly into a chief complaint.

Her phone lights up with overnight MyChart (gl) messages: IUD removal questions. Spotting after a Pap. A possible pregnancy paired with uncertainty. She silences the screen, sits up, and exhales.

Behind her, Malik shifts.

"Clinic day?"

"Clinic day," she answers.

"Save some compassion for home."

"Nurse Practitioner," she corrects automatically, smiling. "But noted."

06:00 — Coffee and the shape of the schedule.

The kettle whistles as dawn arrives. Lena eats yogurt at the counter, tablet propped beside her coffee. The EHR fills in the map of the day: well-woman exams, STI screening, prenatal intake, postpartum mood check, abnormal results.

She scans for red flags — heavy bleeding, severe pain, results discussions, new teen patient — and makes the same promise she makes every morning: listen first, label second.

06:45 — Scrubs, pockets, readiness.

Charcoal scrubs. Sneakers. Hair braided back. She inventories her bag without thinking: Littmann stethoscope, pregnancy wheel (gl), speculum light batteries, patient education pamphlets, protein bar. The cat watches her leave with visible skepticism.

07:25 — Commute through misinformation.

She drives past a mural of women's faces, mentally reviewing screening intervals and HPV (gl) guidelines. A billboard advertising a "Hormone Reset Detox" earns a dramatic eye roll.

She parks as the fog lifts. Another day of untangling bodies from internet myths.

07:50 — Huddle and quiet urgency.

The waiting room is already full — teenagers, couples, women scrolling phones with tight jaws. In huddle, updates stack quickly: prenatal intakes, a colposcopy follow-up, a walk-in for heavy bleeding, supply shortages.

Lena checks her rooms. Speculums. Pap brushes. Swab kits. Doppler (gl). Ready.

08:00 — Well-woman care: autonomy first.

Her first patient is 29, here for an annual exam and oral contraceptive refill (gl).

"I always feel weird being on hormones," the patient says.

Lena explains every step before she does it — breast exam, pelvic exam, Pap smear if due — reminding her she's in control. They talk risks, benefits, alternatives, LARC (gl) options like IUDs and implants, and screening that goes beyond anatomy.

"Your body isn't a problem to manage," Lena says. "It's yours."

"TikTok disagrees," the patient laughs.

"TikTok doesn't bill insurance," Lena replies.

09:15 — Teen visit: safety and agency.

A 16-year-old sits stiffly on the exam table. After confirming confidentiality laws, Lena listens.

A condom broke. The teen didn't know how to get help.

They talk emergency contraception (Plan B) (gl), then long-term options — pill, patch (gl), ring (gl), implant, IUD. Lena screens gently for coercion and safety. The answers are complicated. They often are.

“You’re not in trouble,” Lena says. “You’re taking care of yourself.”

The teen nods, tucking the handout into her hoodie pocket like a secret.

10:30 — Prenatal intake: hope with history.

A couple sits hand-in-hand. First pregnancy to make it this far.

Lena reviews history, orders labs — blood type and Rh (gl), HIV, hepatitis B, rubella immunity (gl) — then rolls in the ultrasound. The room stills.

A flicker appears.

“That’s the heartbeat,” Lena says. “Exactly where we want it.”

She doesn’t promise outcomes. She promises presence.

11:30 — Abnormal results: precision matters.

The Pap shows HSIL (gl) with high-risk HPV (gl). The patient is pale. Google has not been kind.

Lena explains carefully: common virus, precancerous changes, not cancer. Next steps: colposcopy, possible biopsy (gl), maybe LEEP (gl).

“Am I going to die?” the patient asks.

“Not from this,” Lena says firmly. “Not if we follow through. And I’m not leaving you alone with it.”

12:30 — Lunch that isn’t.

Nine minutes. Labs reviewed. Messages sent. A pregnancy with an IUD triggers ectopic pregnancy (gl) alarms. A discreet chlamydia (gl) notification goes out. Sandwich unfinished.

13:00 — Heavy bleeding: not normal.

The add-on patient arrives late, frightened, soaking pads hourly. Lena moves fast: vitals, labs, exam. Fibroids (gl) are likely. Tranexamic acid (gl) started. Ultrasound ordered. Follow-up locked in.

“This is too much bleeding,” Lena says. “We’re not minimizing it.”

14:30 — Postpartum visit: the invisible hemorrhage.

Six weeks post–C-section (gl). Baby sleeping. Mother unraveling.

The physical exam is fine. The mood screen isn’t.

“You’re not broken,” Lena says. “Your brain and body went through an earthquake.” They discuss therapy, support, and starting an SSRI (gl) compatible with breastfeeding.

“You deserve care too.”

16:00 — Closing the loop.

Final visits blur: IUD check (strings visible) (gl), yeast infection (gl), estradiol (gl) refill for a woman reclaiming comfort. Notes finished. Follow-up calls placed.

Lena logs out of Epic, stretches, and exhales.

17:00 — Commute and recalibration.

Golden light. Radio on. The day replays — heartbeats, fear, relief, trust.

18:00 — Home and one sentence.

Leftovers wait. Shoes come off. Later, Lena writes in her journal:

Women's health is never just about organs. It's about power, consent, fear, and futures. My tools are speculums and Pap brushes — but my real job is making sure no one feels dismissed inside their own body.

She closes the notebook. Provider off. Human on.

Chapter 16

Day in the Life — Geriatric Nurse Practitioner

(Community Internal Medicine & Geriatrics Clinic · 08:00–16:30)

05:30 — Old dog, strong coffee, long list.

The coffee pot gurgles in the quiet kitchen. Outside, the sky is still thinking about dawn.

Jonah scratches behind his old lab mix's ears — Sadie grunts in appreciation and flops dramatically back onto her bed.

On the table, his laptop is open to the clinic's EHR schedule:

- Medicare wellness visits.
- Diabetes follow-ups.
- A post-hospital discharge check.
- One slot overbooked for "urgent: dizziness."

He prints his day's list, folds it, and tucks it into his pocket. He knows half of these "15-minute" visits will need twice that. Bodies older than 65 don't respect time slots.

He downs his coffee, slices an apple, and tosses Sadie a treat.

"Geri day, girl," he tells her. "Lots of stories."

She huffs, unimpressed.

06:30 — Commute and med-reconciliation brain.

On the drive, the sun edges over the horizon, turning the freeway orange. Jonah listens to a podcast about polypharmacy (gl) and deprescribing in older adults. He thinks about the patient who came in last month on twelve medications that didn't like each other.

He makes a mental note to check orthostatic vital signs (gl) on anyone with "dizzy" in the chief complaint, and to keep an eye out for the quiet signs of cognitive decline people try to hide.

He parks behind the clinic, stretches his back, and reminds himself: go slow to go fast.

07:45 — Bulletin board, blood pressures, and red flags.

The community clinic shares space with a pharmacy and a physical therapy office. Flyers in the lobby advertise flu shots, balance classes, and bingo night.

"Morning, Jonah," the MA says as he walks in. "Your first three are already here."

He hangs his jacket, logs into Epic, and scans overnight messages: a blood pressure log from a patient trying to avoid adding another medication, a MyChart note from a daughter worried about her dad's memory, a refill request for warfarin (gl) with no recent INR (gl) documented.

He flags the warfarin patient: "Needs INR before refill."

08:00 — Medicare wellness: more than a checklist.

First visit: Mrs. Ramirez, 72, here for her Medicare Annual Wellness Visit (gl). She walks in with a brightly colored tote bag and a stack of papers.

"Thought I'd save you some work," she says, plunking down her home blood pressure log.

Jonah smiles. "You're officially my favorite kind of organized," he says.

They work through the wellness template:

- Height, weight, BMI (gl).
- Vision and hearing screening.
- Fall risk questions.
- Depression screening (PHQ-9) (gl).
- Cognitive screen (Mini-Cog) (gl).

They review her meds, line by line. He asks not just "What do you take?" but "How do you take it?" and "Why do you think you take this one?"

She asks about a weird ad she saw for a supplement. He explains the difference between marketing and evidence, between expensive urine and truly helpful vitamins.

They talk vaccines — pneumococcal (gl), shingles, Tdap (gl) — and advance directives.

"Do you have a living will?" he asks gently.

"My daughter keeps nagging me," she says. "I don't want her to have to decide."

"That's exactly why we talk about it now," he says. "When nobody is in a crisis."

He prints out a packet, promises to go over it with her next visit.

09:00 — Dizziness: between aging and missed diagnoses.

Mr. Brooks, 80, frowns as he sits slowly on the exam table.

"Feels like the room's not where I left it," he says. "Especially when I get up too fast."

The chart says "dizziness." The possibilities in Jonah's mind range from benign positional vertigo to anemia to cardiac arrhythmia to meds.

He starts with orthostatic vitals: lying, sitting, standing blood pressures and heart rates. The MA reads them out — a notable drop when standing; heart rate jumping.

"Let's talk about your meds," Jonah says, moving through the list: beta-blocker (gl), ACE inhibitor (gl), diuretic (gl), something for sleep, something for his prostate.

He does a focused neuro exam, checks for nystagmus (gl), asks about chest pain, shortness of breath, palpitations.

"I think we're overdoing it on your blood pressure meds," Jonah says finally.

They agree to cut back one medication, tighten up hydration, and arrange for a Holter monitor (gl) just to be safe.

10:15 — Diabetes and denial.

Next: 68-year-old man, type 2 diabetes, A1C creeping up despite "mostly" taking his meds.

Jonah reviews labs: A1C 9.2, LDL high, kidney function slightly down.

He checks feet: pulses, sensation with a monofilament (gl), any ulcers lurking between toes.

They adjust meds, adding a GLP-1 agonist (gl) with cardiovascular benefit, and set small, realistic goals.

11:30 — Post-hospital discharge: patching the gaps.

They go through pill bottles: antibiotic? Finish it. New inhaler (gl)? Yes. Duplicate statin? No.

He checks lungs with his stethoscope, reviews warning signs, updates the med list in Epic so it reflects reality.

12:30 — Lunch and lab triage.

Prior auth (gl) frustrations spill over lunch. Labs flag spironolactone (gl) potassium issues, NSAIDs (gl) with ACE inhibitors, anemia hiding behind "just tired."

13:15 — Cognitive changes: between normal aging and something more.

He performs MMSE (gl) and MoCA (gl). Based on history and scores, he suspects early major neurocognitive disorder (dementia) (gl), likely Alzheimer's.

He names it gently and talks safety, resources, and planning.

14:30 — Wounds, warfarin, and walking the line.

INR returns therapeutic. He adjusts dosing, reinforces fall prevention, and prints a clear avoid list.

15:15 — The invisible labor of the last hour.

Home health (gl) orders signed. Mobility device (gl) paperwork completed. Med lists cleaned. Calls made.

16:30 — Charts, then quiet.

He logs out of Epic, stretches, and lets the clinic empty.

18:00 — Old dog, couch, and one sentence.

Later, he writes:

"Geri primary care is slow heroics — catching the medication that causes a fall, naming the memory loss everyone's scared to say out loud, taking enough time with someone that they feel like a person, not a problem list."

Chapter 17

Day in the Life — Emergency Department Nurse Practitioner

(Emergency Department · 11:00–23:00)

08:45 — Blender, headlines, and borrowed calm.

The blender roars over the low murmur of the morning news. Sunlight slices across the kitchen tiles, landing in warm rectangles that Riley's dog, Kona — a lanky husky mix with one blue eye and one brown — keeps pouncing on like they're alive.

Riley pours a blueberry protein smoothie into a tumbler, adds peanut butter toast to the "calories in vs. chaos out" equation, and downs the last of his coffee.

Across the room, his husband, Theo, is already in paramedic (gl) uniform, boots laced, keys in hand.

"Stay safe," Riley calls from the doorway.

"You too, hero," Theo shoots back, half smile, same ritual every shift. Joke, prayer, pact.

Theo leaves; Kona stares at the door, then looks at Riley like, *Your turn.*

Riley props his tablet against the fruit bowl, scrolling through overnight ED notes: boarding patients in hallway beds, a psych hold (gl), an overdose reversal, a stack of "abdominal pain" with vitals that look deceptively normal.

"Full moon energy and it's not even full," he mutters.

He finishes the smoothie, rinses the cup, and tries not to think about how many of those patients are still down there, still waiting.

10:15 — Scrubs, shears, and the go-bag.

Shower steam curls in the bathroom as he mentally runs his checklist: ID badge. Charcoal scrubs. Trauma shears (gl). Penlight. Two pens (one will die by noon). Small notebook. Phone charger. Protein bar. Mask ear savers.

He clips his badge, tucks the trauma shears into a pocket, and gives Kona a final ear scratch.

"Guard the couch," he tells her.

She yawns dramatically. Agreement.

He locks the door and feels the invisible shift: home mode dimming, triage mode booting up.

10:45 — Espresso and sirens.

The city is already loud — food trucks setting up, cyclists weaving through traffic, a siren Doppler-shifting past. He stops at his usual coffee shop.

"Double espresso?" the barista asks.

“ED starter pack,” Riley says.

By the time he pulls into the hospital lot, fatigue has sharpened into focus. The red EMERGENCY sign glows over sliding doors that never really sleep.

10:55 — Into the churn.

The ED hits like weather: fluorescent light, overlapping voices, monitor alarms (gl), the sharp scent of antiseptic layered over sweat and metal.

He scans the tracking board (gl): chest pain, MVC (motor vehicle collision) (gl), laceration, fever, “psych eval,” “feels off.”

“Let’s dance,” he mutters, logging into the EMR.

11:00 — Shift start: inheriting someone else’s storm.

The night NP looks wrecked but wired.

“One admit waiting on a bed. Psych still hasn’t placed the teen in Room 12. Ortho’s late. Two boarders in the hall. STEMI (gl) went to cath. ‘Flu-like’ turned into sepsis.”

“Any time bombs?” Riley asks.

“Chest pains waiting, a febrile infant, and a ‘just not myself’ in six.”

Riley nods. The vague ones are always the loudest in his head.

11:10 — Room 6: chest pain with teeth.

Middle-aged woman, pale, clammy, clutching her chest. The EKG (gl) prints before he even asks. ST elevations.

“This is a heart attack,” he says calmly. “We move fast.”

Aspirin. Nitroglycerin (gl). Heparin (gl). Second IV. Troponin (gl). Activate cath lab (gl).

She squeezes his hand as they wheel her out.

"You're not alone," he tells her.

The room empties. The board fills again.

12:00 — From STEMI to nose treasure.

Room 8 holds a toddler with a purple bead lodged in his nostril and a mother vibrating between panic and rage.

Riley crouches. "We're gonna make the treasure fly."

Positive-pressure (gl). Pop. The bead shoots free. The toddler beams. The mother exhales like she's been underwater.

"Nurse Practitioner," Riley corrects gently when she says doctor. "Same magic. Less debt."

13:00 — The non-TV medicine.

Gallstones (cholelithiasis) (gl). CT scan (gl). Refilled albuterol (gl) for someone who uses the ED as primary care. Hypertension (gl) that never got followed up. Charting between interruptions, thinking three patients ahead while finishing the last one.

Then overhead: *Trauma team to bay one.*

13:45 — Trauma bay: time in snapshots.

MVC rollover. Hypotensive. Femur deformity.

Airway. Breathing. Circulation. FAST exam (gl) positive. Free fluid where it shouldn't be.

"OR now."

Blood. Pressure. Hands moving without conversation. Someone presses a granola bar into his palm afterward. ED love language.

15:00 — Psych is not "attitude."

Teenager. Gown. Sleeves hiding wrists.

"You're not in trouble," Riley says, sitting down.

They talk. About the thought that almost won. About the friend who called 911.

The chart will say *major depressive episode*. Riley will remember it as *someone stayed.*

17:00 — Sutures and jokes.

Box-cutter laceration. Saline (gl). Lidocaine (gl). Interrupted sutures (gl).

"You sew better than my tailor."

"I charge more."

18:45 — Dinner that isn't.

Hummus. Pita. An energy drink he'll regret. A text from Theo.

"You okay?"

"Still breathing. Win."

Pager again: febrile toddler.

19:20 — Racing infection.

Fever 104. Lethargic. Neck stiff.

"Meningitis (gl) is on my list," Riley says calmly.

IV fluids (gl). Blood cultures (gl). Broad-spectrum antibiotics (gl). Coordinating timing for lumbar puncture (gl).

The heart rate settles. Riley doesn't relax, but he breathes.

21:00 — De-escalation in the hallway.

Intoxicated patient. Volume high. Security tense.

"You can yell," Riley says evenly, "or you can get a blanket."

The nervous system settles. No restraints. No tackles. Just containment.

22:00 — The last sprint.

Callbacks. Over-reads (gl). Discharges explained slowly. Hand-offs done carefully.

The EMR shows clicks. It doesn't show the trees he ran through before each decision.

23:05 — Handoff and exhale.

He gives report. Logs out. Board still scrolling. His part done.

23:30 — Wet pavement and quiet.

Rain glistens under streetlights. Riley sits in his car, engine ticking, hands loose on the wheel.

"Twelve hours of borrowed time," he thinks.

00:00 — Couch, dog, husband, silence.

Theo asleep. Kona curled tight. Riley sinks down beside them.

"We both made it," he whispers.

Later, one line in his journal:

Emergency medicine is borrowed time. You push back the worst moments and hope the world gives them another sunrise.

The lights go out. The alarms finally stop.

Chapter 18

Day in the Life — Cardiology Nurse Practitioner

(Cardiac Step-Down Unit · 07:00–15:30)

05:15 — Coffee, rain, and rhythms.

The world outside is all gray and gutters, a slow drizzle making halos around streetlights. Inside the apartment, the air smells like fresh coffee and wet pavement drifting in through a cracked window.

Evan sits at the kitchen table in slate-gray scrubs, bare feet tucked on the chair rung, thumb scrolling through overnight telemetry (gl) reports on his phone. Green squiggles, heart rates, alarms logged and silenced — a chorus of electrical stories.

His husband, Chris, moves around the kitchen in a hoodie and pajama pants, humming as he feeds their orange tabby, Pepper. Pepper meows like a car alarm with fur until the bowl hits the floor.

"Storm's rolling in," Chris says, nodding toward the streaked window. "Good day for hearts to misbehave."

Evan huffs a small laugh. "Good thing I speak fluent arrhythmia."

Breakfast is steel-cut oats, two eggs, half a grapefruit. Cardiologist-approved, NP-enforced.

He closes the telemetry app, sets the phone face up on the table like a promise: these hearts are his to watch for the next eight hours.

Before he leaves, he leans in to kiss Chris, who smells like coffee and dish soap.

"If I'm late, assume somebody's heart had other plans," Evan says.

Chris smiles. "I always do."

06:20 — A soundtrack for systole and diastole.

Rain taps the windshield in steady 4/4 time. Wipers swish, metronome-like. The city is just waking up — buses sighing, taillights stacking in red lines.

Evan queues up Miles Davis, trumpet threading through the gray morning, improvisational and steady at once. It's his pre-round ritual — a reminder that medicine has guidelines, not guarantees.

He thinks of the patients he left yesterday:

• The post-CABG (gl) woman who joked about her "zipper."

• The heart failure (gl) readmit trying not to show how scared he was.

• The older man who cried when he realized he'd survived his second MI (gl).

By the time he pulls into the hospital lot, the last note fades. Cardiology mode clicks on.

06:50 — Badges, beeps, and colored magnets.

He badges into the cardiac step-down unit, where it always smells faintly of coffee, antiseptic, and the ozone tang of old telemetry monitors (gl).

"Morning, NP Evan," the charge nurse calls, surrounded by paper EKG (gl) strips laid out like a paper city.

"You've got a fresh STEMI (gl), a CHF (gl) readmit who thinks 'low salt' means salting once, and your favorite AFib frequent flyer."

Evan steps to the whiteboard. Colored magnets mark each bed: green for stable, yellow for "watch me," red for "don't blink."

Bed 22: post-CABG Day 2 — green-ish.

Bed 24: atrial fibrillation (AFib) (gl) on Cardizem (diltiazem) drip (gl) — yellow.

Bed 26: acute on chronic CHF (gl), being diuresed — yellow-red.

He slings his stethoscope (gl) around his neck and scribbles notes: *22 pain, lungs, ambulation. 24 rate control. 26 daily weights, strict I/O (gl).*

07:00 — Handoff: hearts in summary.

Night shift on one side, day shift on the other, coffee cups forming a defensive line.

"Post-CABG stable. AFib still jumpy. CHF responding to Lasix (furosemide) (gl). New STEMI stented in the LAD — monitor for arrhythmias."

Evan listens, pen moving fast.

"Any chest pain?"

"None post-cath. Family anxious."

Information files into mental drawers labeled *Immediate*, *Watch*, *Don't Forget*.

07:20 — Rounds: translating electricity into plans.

The cardiology team moves room to room, decisions stacking quickly.

At Bed 22, Mrs. Tanaka smiles.

"How's the new plumbing?" Evan asks.

"Louder than my husband."

Heart steady. Lungs clear enough. Legs without edema (gl).

"Schedule Tylenol (gl). PRN oxycodone (gl) backup. CXR (gl) later. Lasix early."

At Bed 24, the monitor flickers with AFib.

"Cardizem drip at ten."

"BP?"

"118/72."

"Bolus ten. Let's aim for the 90s."

Orders in. Team moves.

08:30 — Post-op check: zippered chest, steady rhythm.

Evan listens carefully. Regular rhythm. Minimal basilar crackles (gl). No pitting edema.

"We'll keep the ACE inhibitor (gl) and beta-blocker (gl) on board," he says. "Keep that EF (gl) happy."

She rolls her eyes at PT. He grins and updates Epic (gl): *Excellent rehab candidate.*

09:10 — Telemetry city.

Night strips wait like a skyline.

AFib runs. Benign PVCs (gl). A brief nonsustained VT (gl) post-cath.

"Flag Bed 28 for EP (electrophysiology)," Evan says.

Coffee goes cold. He drinks it anyway.

10:00 — Family meeting: explaining a tired heart.

Echo (echocardiogram) (gl) report folded between them.

"Your dad's heart isn't squeezing as strongly," Evan explains, sketching chambers. "The ejection fraction (EF) (gl) is low."

"Can you fix it?"

"We can help it work better."

Meds. Sodium restriction (gl). Daily weights. Time.

"We don't forget there's a person attached to every EF."

Fear settles into understanding.

10:45 — Inbox storm.

Refills. Labs. BNP (gl). Potassium (gl) low. Old troponin alerts screaming anyway.

He answers quickly, clearly, kindly.

“Survival,” he tells the resident eyeing his granola bar.

11:15 — Discharge teaching: meds and metaphors.

ACE inhibitor (gl). Beta-blocker (gl). Diuretic (gl). Statin (gl). Aspirin (gl).

Nitroglycerin (gl) goes under the tongue — not in a glove box.

He highlights, prints, and sends a summary to primary care. Redundancy is care.

12:30 — Lunch and rain-streaked windows.

Pretzels labeled “low-sodium rebels only.” Half a sandwich gone when the pager vibrates.

AFib with RVR (gl). Lunch ends.

13:00 — Alarm: AFib speeds up.

Rate 150. Cardizem bolus (gl). Fresh EKG (gl).

Heart rate drifts down.

“Nah,” Evan says. “Not on my watch.”

13:40 — Echo lab: watching a tired pump work.

Mild mitral regurgitation (gl). No change today.

The heart keeps squeezing because it doesn't know how to quit.

14:30 — The favorite survivor.

"Worth every beat," Mr. Dunbar says.

Rhythm steady. No ischemia. More hallway laps.

15:00 — The invisible density of the last hour.

Calls. Corrections. Potassium replacement (gl). Telemetry sign-offs.

A note for night shift: *BP trend worries me.*

15:40 — Drive home under a clearing sky.

Rain softens. Miles Davis returns.

Today, several hearts got another chance.

16:10 — Home: art supplies and a cat who doesn't care about EF.

Dinner, laughter, no alarms. Pepper knocks something off the counter for sport.

21:00 — Nightly reflection: time kept in beats.

Evan writes:

Hearts remember trauma, forgive late changes, and keep time for stories still being told.

Tomorrow: new names, new rhythms.

Same work — catching stutters, smoothing chaos, honoring the organ that refuses to quit.

Chapter 19

Day in the Life — Neonatal Nurse Practitioner

(NICU | 06:30–18:30)

04:45 — Kettle, glow, and grams

The kettle clicks on in the dark, a small sound in a house still asleep. Camila moves through the kitchen by muscle memory alone: green tea into the infuser, bread into the toaster, phone unlocked to the NICU app before the water even boils.

Two new admissions overnight. One stable preterm infant. One vented with rising oxygen needs. Her thumb scrolls through gestational ages, birth weights, and FiO_2 (gl) settings — decimals that translate into risk, vigilance, and hope.

Upstairs, her wife Harper sleeps beside the baby monitor, the soft hiss of their three-month-old's breathing filling the room. Camila spreads peanut butter on toast, glances at the monitor, and smiles.

"You're the only preemie I visit who yells when I leave," she murmurs.

She eats standing up, tea cooling beside her, absorbing the overnight handoff before the day has officially begun.

05:15 — Scrubs, badge, and one more crib check

The shower is quick. Hair pulled tight. Periwinkle scrubs embroidered with *Camila R., NNP-BC*. Badge clipped beside a small rainbow pin.

Before heading out, she pauses at Lily's crib. The baby sleeps sprawled, one fist curled near her mouth.

"Be good for Mama," Camila whispers. "I'm going to help some other tiny fighters today."

Harper mumbles encouragement from the bed. Camila grabs her lunch — yogurt, salad, a granola bar she'll eat between alarms — and steps into the dark.

05:45 — The drive: quiet before the beeps

The roads are empty, dawn just beginning to stretch pink across the sky. Camila drives in silence, already rounding in her head.

Who's on CPAP (gl). Who's on high-flow nasal cannula (gl). Who might tolerate weaning phototherapy (gl) today.

The two new admits replay in her mind: a 29-weeker at 1,220 grams on CPAP, a 32-weeker on TPN (gl) with borderline sugars.

By the time she parks, she's already handed herself the morning.

06:20 — Stepping into the womb of the hospital

The NICU doors slide open with a soft hiss. Warm, humid air replaces the hallway chill.

Isolettes (gl) line the unit in neat rows. Monitors glow blue and green. Ventilators (gl) sigh. Infusion pumps (gl) tick steadily.

"Morning, Camila," the charge nurse whispers. Voices are always softer here, as if sound itself could startle fragile lungs.

Camila sets down her bag and reaches for the handoff sheet.

06:30 — Handoff: grams, sats, and small miracles

The night NNP runs down the list.

"Baby A weaned on CPAP overnight. FiO_2 down to thirty. Baby C had a few desats (gl), self-resolved. Baby L still on high-frequency oscillatory ventilation (gl), gases improving."

Two new admits. One sugar watch. One long day already in motion.

Each line on the whiteboard is a life suspended between too early and just enough.

07:00 — Morning rounds: milliliters and restraint

Rounds move bedspace to bedspace — neonatologist, nurses, respiratory therapist, pharmacist.

"Feeds at fifteen milliliters every three hours," a nurse reports.

"Advance to eighteen," Camila says. "Fortify to twenty-four calories. Hold phototherapy if bilirubin stays down."

At the ventilated infant's bedside, she studies numbers that demand patience.

“No sudden moves,” she says quietly. “This one’s a long game.”

Every order sounds small. None of them are.

08:15 — Hands gentle, eyes fierce

Camila adjusts CPAP prongs on a baby whose entire head fits in her palm. Skin checks. Positioning. Always prevention before rescue.

Nearby, a nurse changes a diaper smaller than Camila’s hand.

“Best part of the job,” Camila murmurs, watching.

09:30 — New admit: 29 weeks and brand-new

The transport team arrives with a transport isolette (gl), cords and tubes framing a body barely bigger than Camila’s forearm.

“Brief positive pressure at birth,” the nurse reports. “Now stable on CPAP.”

Camila takes the lead, voice calm and deliberate.

“Warm, dry, stimulate. Switch to our circuit. Start caffeine (gl). Check glucose — D10 (gl) if needed.”

When the baby settles under the warmer, she exhales.

“He’s here,” she says. “He’s ours.”

10:45 — Charting, coffee, and translation

Camila logs into Epic (gl), documenting feeds, labs, parental updates. Coffee tastes burnt. She drinks it anyway.

When parents ask for updates, she swaps clinical precision for clarity.

"He gained twenty grams," she tells them. "That's huge at his size."

They cry. In the NICU, grams matter.

11:15 — Family conference: redefining progress

A young couple sits across from her, fear heavy in the room.

She explains IVH (gl) risks and ROP (gl) screening without catastrophizing.

"We celebrate grams and minutes," she says. "We don't rush the future."

They leave steadier than they arrived.

12:30 — Lunch and coping rituals

Cookies shaped like baby footprints sit on the counter.

"We cope weirdly," a nurse says.

Camila eats one. Guidelines scroll on her phone. Work never fully leaves.

13:10 — Alarm: apnea

A monitor shrills.

"Apnea (gl)," someone calls.

Camila is already there, rubbing a tiny back until breathing returns.

"Adjust FiO_2 five percent," she says. "Check caffeine timing."

Her pulse settles last.

14:00 — Ultrasound rounds

Head ultrasound (gl) screens glow in grayscale.

"No bleed," the radiologist says.

Camila feels relief move through her shoulders. Wins are quiet here.

15:00 — Micro-care, macro meaning

She changes a diaper on a twenty-five-weeker, movements slow, deliberate.

Every touch teaches safety.

16:45 — Evening weans and careful optimism

TPN adjusted. Labs reviewed. Parents called.

"Thirty grams today," she tells one family. "That's progress."

She leaves meticulous handoff notes. Night shift will inherit everything.

18:10 — Handoff and lullaby beeps

The unit dims. Voices soften.

CPAP. HFNC. Who needs clustered care. Who needs extra explanation.

The monitors hum their coded lullaby.

18:45 — Drive home

Sunlight turns gold. The hospital fades. The babies do not.

19:10 — Home: another kind of NICU

Lily grabs her badge and laughs.

"You're my toughest patient," Camila says.

Normal life resumes. It has to.

21:00 — Miracles in milliliters

Later, she writes:

"In the NICU, miracles are measured in grams. The goal is not survival alone, but a life that gets to forget how close it came."

She turns out the light, ready to do it all again tomorrow.

Chapter 20

Day in the Life — Psychiatric Nurse Practitioner

(Outpatient Behavioral Health Clinic | 09:00–17:30)

06:45 — Coffee, headlines, and calibrated concern

The coffee machine hisses in an otherwise quiet kitchen. Outside, early light washes the street in gray-blue, a jogger passing with reflective bands blinking like distant signals.

Ava stirs almond milk into her mug and scrolls through the news. Another grim headline. Another reminder of why her waiting room never empties.

She flips the phone face down. She doesn't need more evidence that the world is anxious.

Across the table, her partner Lina — a social worker — is already dressed, laptop open, calendar crowded with home visits and school meetings.

"Big day?" Lina asks.

"Eight follow-ups, three intakes," Ava says. "One court-mandated anger referral. One medication-resistant depression. One teenager whose mother emailed in all caps."

"So... a normal Tuesday," Lina says.

Ava smiles, then glances at her notebook, where she keeps grounding reminders: *Hold space. Ask one more question. Check the meds — and the story.*

07:30 — Commute and cognitive warm-up

On the train, Ava sits by the window, earbuds in, letting music soften the clatter. She reviews notes from a recent continuing education (gl) session on SSRI switching strategies and newer data on ketamine (gl) for treatment-resistant depression.

Patients move through her mind in shorthand: benzodiazepine tapers (gl), postpartum depression tangled with stigma, a nonbinary teen navigating anxiety and identity at once.

The science matters. So does how you ask, *How are you really?* without turning someone into a problem to be solved.

08:45 — Waiting room energy

The clinic sits on the fifth floor of a glass office building — more law firms than hospitals in view.

Inside, the waiting room is intentionally soft: muted colors, low shelves, no televisions blaring bad news. A white-noise machine hums gently.

"Your nine o'clock is here," the front-desk coordinator says. "Your nine-thirty is early. And your ten has already called twice."

Ava scans the schedule in the EHR (gl), then steps into her office — two armchairs, a desk, a worn rug, a tissue box that never stays full.

She logs in, reviews medications, labs, prior notes, and reminds herself: no one is just their diagnosis.

09:00 — Follow-up: 'I'm fine' and what it hides

Mark, a 42-year-old software engineer with major depressive disorder (gl), sits stiffly, arms folded.

"How've you been?" Ava asks.

"I'm fine," he says automatically.

She waits. Silence does some of the work for her.

Sleep is fragmented. Energy is low. Concentration unreliable. He admits he's been skipping SSRI doses because it "doesn't feel like it's doing anything" and drinking more than he planned.

They talk adherence, expectations, and the difference between *partial response* and *no response*. They agree on a cautious dose increase and closer follow-up, with therapy frequency reinforced.

"Depression lies," Ava says. "It tells you nothing will help so you won't try what might."

He smiles despite himself.

Her note reads: *Partial response, adherence issues addressed, med adjusted, no acute SI.*

Her internal note is shorter: *Check in sooner.*

09:45 — Intake: panic in a teenager's body

Sixteen-year-old Layla sits rigidly beside her mother, eyes fixed on the carpet. Referral: panic attacks at school.

Ava asks Mom to step out briefly. Alone, the room feels smaller.

Layla describes racing heart, chest pain, tingling hands — panic disorder (gl) by the book. Ava screens carefully for medical contributors, depression, suicidal ideation.

They talk psychoeducation (gl): fight-or-flight, adrenaline, why breathing exercises aren't pointless but physiological retraining.

A low-dose SSRI is started. Therapy is emphasized as essential, not optional. They practice box breathing (gl) until Layla feels her heart slow.

"You're not broken," Ava says. "Your alarm system is just loud. We can teach it when to stand down."

Layla nods, fear still present, but less alone.

11:00 — Medication management: language, stigma, side effects

A 55-year-old woman with bipolar II disorder (gl) wants to stop her atypical antipsychotic (gl).

"I hate that word," she says. "And I feel foggy."

They review side effects and revisit life before stabilization — impulsivity, hypomania, depressive crashes.

"Medication names are outdated," Ava says. "They don't define you. They're tools."

They agree on a cautious dose reduction with close monitoring. Safety is explicit. Nothing is rushed.

The note reflects both: *Distress about side effects and labeling. Plan adjusted. Monitoring emphasized.*

12:30 — Lunch and system friction

In the break room, someone vents about prior authorization delays for an SNRI (gl).

"They want three failures first," a colleague says.

Ava eats soup while finishing notes, messaging therapists, reviewing labs (gl) that masquerade as psychiatric symptoms.

A low TSH (gl) flags in a patient with new-onset anxiety. She messages the PCP. Mental health does not exist in isolation.

13:15 — Court-mandated anger

A 28-year-old man sits slouched, arms crossed.

"I'm only here so they'll drop the charges," he says.

Ava nods. "That's fine. While you're here, we can talk about why your body goes straight to fight mode."

History reveals trauma, poor sleep, heavy alcohol use. She screens for PTSD (gl), substance use disorder, depression.

She doesn't moralize. She contextualizes.

They discuss anger management therapy (gl) and possible pharmacologic support for irritability.

Goal #1 goes in the chart verbatim: *Avoid re-arrest.*

14:30 — Treatment-resistant depression

Her most complex visit of the day. A woman exhausted by years of medication trials.

“I’m tired of being the experiment,” the patient says.

“You’re not,” Ava replies. “The meds are.”

They review augmentation strategies (gl), TMS (gl), and referral for ketamine (gl) evaluation. Safety is reassessed carefully. Passive SI is acknowledged, not dramatized.

“We’re building a net,” Ava says. “I’m not going anywhere.”

The plan is conservative. The follow-up is sooner than standard.

16:00 — Identity, recovery, and executive function

The final stretch brings variety:

• A nonbinary teen adjusting to sertraline (gl), anxiety intertwined with dysphoria (gl).

• A man celebrating sixty days sober, discussing naltrexone (gl).

• A graduate student navigating ADHD and stimulant (gl) initiation with structure and safeguards.

Each visit ends with the same permission: *You’re allowed to need something different later.*

17:30 — Closure without resolution

Ava finishes her last note, returns a therapist’s call, answers a patient portal message that reads, *Other people have it worse.*

Her reply is brief: *Pain isn’t a competition. Yours counts.*

She logs out, turns off the light, and walks past an empty waiting room.

18:15 — Commute home

On the train, she resists reading more studies. She lets the day settle.

Not weights — postcards. Proof people showed up.

19:00 — Ordinary life

Dinner, dishes, small complaints about plumbing. Problems with solutions. It feels luxurious.

22:00 — One line to hold the day

In bed, Ava writes one sentence:

"Psychiatry is staying long enough that someone remembers they are not the worst thought they've ever had."

She turns out the light.

Tomorrow will bring new names, familiar diagnoses, and different stories.

Same work: believing people until they can borrow that belief back.

SCRUB*fits*™ Reflection — Anna Remedy, DNP, FNP-BC, PMHNP

"One of the most important questions to ask after reading a day like this is not whether you could perform the work, but whether the pace, responsibility, and decision-making rhythm feel sustainable for you over time. Nurse Practitioner practice often rewards people who are comfortable carrying

independent clinical judgment while still working inside team-based systems. If the balance of autonomy, accountability, and patient continuity you saw in this chapter feels energizing, that signal matters. If it feels heavy or draining, that signal matters just as much. Alignment is not about capability — it is about sustainability."

Chapter 21

Day in the Life — Virtual Nurse Practitioner

(Care Through a Screen, Connection Through Presence)

06:27 — Waking Up in a House That Is Also a Clinic

The house is quiet in the particular way it only is before the day asserts itself. Morning light slips through the curtains in pale bands as Jordan wakes, stretching slowly, already aware of the strange duality ahead.

This is the paradox of virtual care: work exists ten steps away, close enough to feel efficient, close enough to blur boundaries if you let it.

His golden retriever, Maple, thumps her tail against the bed frame. She knows the rhythm of his mornings—breakfast first, laptop second, walk postponed until later.

Jordan moves into the kitchen, making oatmeal and coffee with the deliberate gentleness of someone who cannot afford to start the day rushed. He opens the back door and Maple bolts into the yard, conducting her daily perimeter sweep as if defending against invisible threats. Leaves. Squirrels. Wind.

Jordan leans against the doorframe, mug warm in his hands, breathing in the cool air. Telehealth demands presence. Presence requires arriving fully, even when you never leave the house.

07:11 — Preparing the Virtual Clinic

His home office is spare but intentional. A ring light angled to avoid shadows. Neutral greenery behind him. Diplomas placed just within frame—credibility without performance. A noise-canceling microphone. A second monitor. A secure Wi-Fi connection with a backup hotspot already tested.

This is not casual medicine. It is infrastructure.

He logs into the EHR and scans the day's schedule: twenty-two patients. Acute visits. Chronic disease follow-ups. Behavioral health check-ins. A few visits that will end in reassurance, a few that will demand decisiveness, and several that will be more complicated than the reason listed.

Morning labs populate the screen—A1Cs, lipid panels, thyroid results, photos uploaded overnight with messages that read *Does this look normal?* It rarely does.

A secure message appears from the medical assistant:

Your first patient is early and very anxious.

Jordan exhales once, slow and deliberate. Telehealth isn't clicking boxes. It's reading energy through a screen.

08:00 — Visit One: Anxiety With a Side of Technology

The woman appears pixelated, the image unstable, her voice breaking in and out.

“Can you hear me? I don’t think my mic—hold on—wait—”

Jordan keeps his tone calm and steady, guiding her through the basics. Click here. Try that. It takes a minute, but when the sound stabilizes, she exhales audibly, shoulders dropping.

Sometimes the first treatment is simply being heard.

They talk through her symptoms—panic episodes, insomnia, chest tightness. Jordan watches her hands, tapping just out of frame. He asks her to hold the pill bottle up to the camera. Sertraline. Low dose. Recently started.

They discuss side effects, expectations, and next steps. A cautious dose increase. Grounding strategies. A follow-up sooner than scheduled.

Before the visit ends, she says quietly, “Thank you for not making me feel stupid.”

Jordan meets her eyes through the screen. “Nothing about anxiety is stupid.”

08:28 — Visit Two: Pink Eye, Probably

A father joins holding a toddler who clearly does not consent to being examined. The child wriggles, attempting escape while the father apologizes repeatedly.

Jordan laughs—an essential telehealth skill.

With parent-assisted assessment, the picture becomes clear. Redness. Discharge. Crusting.

Conjunctivitis.

He sends the prescription, reviews hygiene, reassures the father, and ends the visit as the toddler attempts to lick the camera lens. Some parts of primary care are universal.

09:14 — Chronic Disease, Creative Care

Mr. Harrell logs in smiling, glucose logs already pulled up. Type 2 diabetes. Hypertension. Humor as a coping strategy.

They review numbers, adjust medications, talk through foot care.

“Can you angle the camera down a bit?” Jordan asks.

The image shifts. Skin looks intact. Nails trimmed. Not perfect —but sufficient.

“You’re my favorite computer doctor,” Mr. Harrell says.

Jordan takes the compliment.

10:52 — The Technology Wall

Mid-morning brings predictable chaos. Frozen screens. Audio loops. Patients talking into the wrong microphone. One visit conducted from a parked car outside a fast-food restaurant.

Telehealth is part medicine, part improvisation, part customer support.

Jordan stays patient. Frustration never helps the connection.

11:30 — Lunch Without a Pause

Leftovers go into the microwave. Secure messages pile up before the first bite. Refill requests. Work notes. Symptom photos.

He eats anyway. Telehealth lunches are functional, not restorative.

12:10 — The Lonely Visit

An older woman logs in. Mild hypertension. Stable labs. The visit stretches gently beyond its medical purpose.

"I'm glad to see you," she says.

Jordan means it when he replies, "I'm glad to see you too."

Not every encounter needs medication. Sometimes presence is the intervention.

13:50 — Dermatology by Camera

A young man holds his phone inches from his forearm. Red. Itchy. Expanding.

Jordan guides him through lighting, distance, and angle adjustments. The diagnosis becomes clear enough to act. Treatment is straightforward. Education included.

Telehealth rewards clinicians who can tolerate imperfection without sacrificing safety.

15:11 — Work Note Negotiations

A patient asks for four days off for mild symptoms.

Jordan assesses carefully. No red flags. No justification for extended leave.

He provides a note for today.

Boundaries are part of care—for the patient and the clinician.

16:46 — The Emotional Weight of the Day

Postpartum depression fills the screen. Dark circles. Quiet distress.

Jordan slows everything down. Adjusts medication. Discusses sleep strategies. Reinforces support. No multitasking. No rushing.

Telehealth becomes a lifeline for patients who cannot leave home—and for clinicians willing to stay present through a screen.

18:02 — Logging Out

Jordan finishes charting, clears the inbox, and logs out. He sits still for a moment, letting the silence settle.

Virtual care looks gentle from the outside. It is not. It requires sustained attention, emotional availability, and deliberate boundaries.

18:28 — Re-Entering Life

He closes the office door. Maple reappears instantly, tail spinning.

Lila hands him tea. "How was it?"

"Good," he says. "Humans are complicated. Technology even more so."

Tomorrow will bring more screens, more connection, more unpredictability.

Tonight is for rest.

SCRUB*fits*™ Reflection — Anna Remedy, DNP, FNP-BC, PMHNP

"Virtual Nurse Practitioner roles change the rhythm of clinical interaction. Without the traditional exam room, communication skills, listening precision, and clinical judgment become even more central to effective care. Some clinicians appreciate the focused, technology-enabled workflow, while others miss the physical presence of in-person encounters. Alignment in telehealth often depends less on technology comfort and more on whether virtual patient relationships feel meaningful and sustainable to you."

Chapter 22

Day in the Life — Neurology Nurse Practitioner

(Comprehensive Stroke & Epilepsy Center | 07:00–17:00)

04:45 — Alarm, aura, and anticipation

The alarm cuts through the dark before dawn. Malik lies still for a moment, already mapping the day ahead: stroke alerts, seizure follow-ups, medication adjustments, MRI results that will quietly redraw people's futures. Neurology does not wait for full daylight.

Beside him, his partner Dev rolls over. "Brains today?" he asks, half-asleep.

"When is it not brains?" Malik replies, leaning down to kiss his forehead. "Go back to sleep. I'll bring pastries tomorrow."

In the kitchen, coffee pours while Malik scrolls through overnight pages on his phone. A stroke code at 02:10. tPA (gl) administered. ICU admission. An Epilepsy Monitoring Unit (EMU) (gl) patient with breakthrough seizures. A clinic message about a new hand tremor.

The weight settles in. Brains don't rest. Neither does neurology.

05:30 — Breakfast and brain maps

Eggs sizzle. Sourdough toasts. Avocado makes a deliberate appearance, like an offering to preventive medicine. Malik flips through a pocket reference while he eats: updated American Heart Association/American Stroke Association (AHA/ASA) (gl) stroke guidance, new data on direct oral anticoagulants (DOACs) (gl), recent changes in anti-seizure medications (gl).

He thinks of yesterday's patient who said, "I feel like my brain betrayed me," after seizing on a crowded subway platform.

He rinses his mug, clips on his badge, and steps into the early morning.

06:20 — Commute and cranial nerves

The highway is mostly empty. Malik reviews cranial nerves (gl) in his head, not because he needs to, but because neurology rewards precision.

I — smell.

II — vision.

III, IV, VI — eye movements.

V — facial sensation.

VII — facial expression.

Details are lives.

06:50 — Monitors, MRI lists, and morning huddle

The neurology floor hums with its familiar low urgency. Central monitors flicker. A whiteboard lists beds and diagnoses: stroke (gl), seizure, Guillain-Barré syndrome (gl), multiple sclerosis (gl), rule-out TIA (transient ischemic attack) (gl).

"Morning, NP Malik," the charge nurse calls. "Stroke team huddle in five. EMU was busy."

He logs into Epic (gl), reviews his inpatient list, and joins the huddle. Overnight events are rapid-fire: a post-tPA patient improving, a new-onset seizure with abnormal EEG (gl), pending MRIs stacked like unanswered questions.

"NIHSS (gl) dropped from twelve to four," the resident reports on the stroke patient.

Malik nods. Good signs — but not permission to relax.

07:30 — Stroke rounds: seconds and synapses

Bed eight. The man who arrived aphasic and weak now lifts both arms on command. There is still drift on the right, but it is subtle. Encouraging.

Malik moves through the NIH Stroke Scale (gl) methodically — gaze, fields, facial movement, motor strength, sensation, language, neglect.

"Significant improvement," he tells the attending. "We'll monitor closely for hemorrhagic transformation, but this looks like a strong tPA response."

They outline the next steps: MRI brain (gl), magnetic resonance angiography (MRA) (gl), echocardiogram (gl), anticoagulation decisions depending on rhythm monitoring.

To the patient and family, Malik translates: "The clot-busting medication worked. Now our job is figuring out why this happened — and preventing it from happening again."

09:00 — EMU: seizures on screen

In the EMU, EEG caps (gl) and cameras surround patients whose brains are being asked to reveal their secrets.

Emma, twenty-seven, hasn't slept well.

Her overnight EEG (gl) captured a seizure — rhythmic sharp activity in the left temporal region.

"So... they're real?" she asks quietly.

"They're real," Malik says. "Not imagined. Not exaggerated. A real electrical problem in the brain."

They discuss switching from levetiracetam (gl), which has worsened her mood, to lamotrigine (gl), reviewing slow titration and serious rash risks like Stevens-Johnson syndrome (gl). Seizure precautions are clear. No sugarcoating, no catastrophizing.

"You're not broken," Malik tells her. "Your brain is misfiring. We can work with that."

10:30 — Clinic: detective work in motion

The morning clinic brings familiar complexity. A woman with chronic migraine (gl) who has tried triptans (gl), beta-blockers (gl), magnesium (gl), and patience. Malik reviews her headache diary, screens for medication overuse (gl), and discusses newer options: CGRP monoclonal antibodies (gl), Botox (gl), and lifestyle levers that actually matter.

"We can't make your brain forget migraines exist," he says. "But we can reduce how often it chooses them."

Next, a fifty-two-year-old with hand numbness. Malik works through the differential: carpal tunnel syndrome (gl), peripheral neuropathy (gl), cervical radiculopathy (gl). His exam is deliberate — reflexes, sensation, Tinel's sign (gl), Phalen's test (gl).

The plan includes nerve conduction studies (NCS/EMG) (gl), wrist splints, and coordination with primary care for glycemic control.

12:30 — Lunch and lesions

He eats quickly while reviewing MRI reports: new enhancing lesion in periventricular white matter. No acute infarct. Multifocal microbleeds.

He flags an MS patient for possible escalation of disease-modifying therapy (DMT) (gl).

A worried patient calls about "brain spots." Malik explains white matter hyperintensities (gl) in plain language.

"MRI machines see everything," he says. "Our job is deciding what matters."

13:30 — MS follow-up: living with uncertainty

Alicia, thirty-one, has relapsing-remitting multiple sclerosis (RRMS) (gl). Her scans are stable. Her fatigue is not.

They talk honestly about energy limits, medication timing, vitamin D (gl), and whether agents like amantadine (gl) or modafinil (gl) might help. Physical and occupational therapy referrals focus on conserving energy, not forcing endurance.

"You're allowed to be frustrated with your nervous system," Malik says. "That doesn't mean you're failing."

15:00 — Stroke in real time

A sudden page: facial droop in the waiting room. Stroke code activated.

Malik moves fast. Exam. NIHSS (gl) around eight. Blood glucose normal. CT head (gl) negative for bleed. CT angiography (CTA) (gl) reveals a left middle cerebral artery (MCA) (gl) branch occlusion.

He explains tPA (alteplase) (gl) risks and benefits clearly: percentages, outcomes, urgency without panic. Consent is given. The infusion begins.

Minutes later, the patient's hand moves more easily. A corner of the mouth lifts.

The room exhales.

16:30 — Cognitive residue

The final hour is documentation and coordination. Calls to families. Messages to therapy teams. Notes that must be exact.

He types until the screen blurs slightly: stroke care, epilepsy management, migraine plans. He logs out of Epic (gl) feeling drained and alert at the same time — neurology's particular aftertaste.

17:30 — Deceleration

Driving home, Malik lets music pull him out of diagnostic

mode. The day replays anyway: EEG spikes, Doppler waveforms, fingers moving again after paralysis.

18:00 — One sentence to hold it all

At home, curry waits. Dev asks, "How were the neurons?"

"Dramatic," Malik says. "But cooperative."

Later, he writes one line in his journal:

"Neurology is listening to electricity tell stories — and sometimes, if you arrive fast enough, you get to change the ending."

Tomorrow will bring new scans, new seizures, new strokes.

Same work: guarding the brain's fragile current.

SCRUB*fits*™ Reflection — Anna Remedy, DNP, FNP-BC, PMHNP

"Neurology Nurse Practitioner practice allows deeper expertise in a focused clinical area, often bringing more predictable patient populations and highly specialized workflows. Many clinicians enjoy mastering a defined domain, while others eventually miss the variety found in broader practice settings. Consider whether depth or variety tends to keep you engaged over time. Long-term satisfaction often follows the environments where curiosity remains active."

Chapter 23

Day in the Life — Dermatology Nurse Practitioner

(Outpatient Skin Cancer & Medical Dermatology Clinic | 08:00–18:00)

06:30 — Sunrise, SPF, and skin in the mirror

Leah wakes before her alarm, early light edging around the blackout curtains. Years in dermatology have turned her morning routine into a quiet public service announcement. She splashes cool water on her face, pats dry, and reaches automatically for broad-spectrum sunscreen (gl), working it into her cheeks, forehead, neck, and the backs of her hands.

In the mirror, she notices a light scatter of freckles across her nose from last weekend's hike. "You know better," she murmurs, half amused, half stern. Her eyes drift to the small scar on her left shoulder where her own dermatologist biopsied a mole last year — benign, but still capable of making her pulse jump for a second.

Coffee brews while she scrolls through the day's schedule: full-body skin exams, acne follow-ups, biologic (gl) injections for psoriasis (gl), and several visits flagged as "rule-out melanoma (gl), very worried." The worry is rarely about the lesion alone; it's about how long someone has been staring at it in the mirror, imagining outcomes.

Her partner, Miguel, wanders in, hair still flattened by sleep.

"Sunscreen sermon today?" he asks, reaching for the French press.

"Always," Leah says. "I make a living nagging people into keeping their epidermis (gl) intact and unmutated."

He grins, kisses her temple, and nods at her hands. "You missed a spot."

She sighs, pumps more SPF, and they laugh.

07:35 — Commute and mental mapping

Traffic is light. Leah drives in silence, running through the day ahead: the older farmer with a non-healing ear lesion; the teenager starting isotretinoin (gl) for severe cystic acne (gl); the teacher anxious about switching to injectable therapy; the young woman who noticed an asymmetrical mole during pregnancy.

Her mind cycles through the quiet frameworks dermatology runs on: the ABCDEs of melanoma (gl); the clinical differences between basal cell carcinoma (gl) and squamous cell carcinoma (gl); when a shave biopsy (gl) is enough and when a punch biopsy (gl) is smarter; how often a "rash" turns out to be a medication reaction rather than eczema.

She parks under the single strip of shade in the lot, grabs her lunch, and heads inside past the clinic's glass front and its cheerful metal sun sculpture — beloved by patients, quietly resented by staff.

07:55 — Pre-clinic huddle: spots, slots, and frozen nitrogen

In the staff room, Dr. Ahmed reviews the schedule with Leah and the medical assistants. The liquid nitrogen (gl) canister hisses softly in the corner.

“We’ve got urgent mole slots this morning,” he says, tapping the screen, “a high-risk full-body exam, and a couple of post-Mohs surgery (gl) wound checks.”

“Room three is set for biopsies,” the charge MA adds. “We’re short one MA this afternoon, so turnover needs to be tight.”

Leah nods. “I’ll take the isotretinoin consults and the fungal follow-ups. They’ll come with questions.”

They review safety checks — allergies, emergency medications, epinephrine (gl) availability — and then the doors open.

08:15 — Full-body skin exam: scars and sun histories

Susan, sixty-three, sits on the exam table in a paper gown, fingers worrying the edge. A melanoma was removed from her calf three years ago. Annual exams still carry weight.

“Anything new or changing?” Leah asks, rolling closer.

Susan points to her upper arm. “This one. My husband says it’s nothing. The internet says it’s everything.”

Leah smiles. “Let’s ask the dermatoscope (gl).”

She works methodically — scalp to soles — narrating as she goes so Susan never feels examined in silence. Seborrheic keratoses (gl). Cherry angiomas (gl). Benign, common, unthreatening.

When she reaches the mole Susan flagged, Leah pauses. Asymmetry. Varied pigmentation. Nothing dramatic, but enough.

"I'm not alarmed," Leah says, meeting her eyes, "but I don't like guessing. This one earns a biopsy."

She explains the shave biopsy: lidocaine (gl), quick removal, aluminum chloride (gl) for hemostasis, bandage. Susan exhales as the sting fades.

"In dermatology," Leah says, labeling the specimen, "tiny samples tell us big truths."

They finish with aftercare, sunscreen counseling, and permission to live normally without fear of the sun.

09:30 — Acne and identity: isotretinoin conversations

Jayden, seventeen, sits curled into himself, hood pulled low despite the warm room. His cystic acne is painful and already scarring.

Leah angles her stool sideways, meeting him at shoulder level.

"What's your skin been like lately?"

"Bad," he says.

"What does 'bad' mean for you?"

"It hurts. People stare. I avoid pictures."

They've exhausted reasonable first-line treatments. Today is the isotretinoin conversation.

Leah uses a simple diagram. "This medication turns down the oil production that feeds these cysts. It's powerful, so we respect it — labs, monitoring, regular visits."

She reviews side effects clearly and without drama, screens for mood symptoms, and acknowledges the emotional toll of visible disease.

"What do you want your face to feel like in six months?" she asks.

Jayden thinks. "Like something I don't think about all day."

"That's a goal worth working toward."

They enroll in the safety monitoring program (gl), set expectations, and build a simple skin-care plan. As he leaves, Jayden murmurs, "Thanks for not making me take the hoodie off right away."

"I go at your pace," Leah replies. "Skin is attached to a person."

11:00 — The 'weird rash' that isn't simple

Mrs. Patel lifts her sari hem to reveal symmetrical, scaly plaques around both ankles. Over-the-counter creams haven't helped.

Leah studies the distribution, checks nails and scalp, and listens to the story. Nail pitting. Subtle scalp involvement. This isn't eczema (gl).

"This looks more like psoriasis," Leah explains. "Your immune system is telling skin cells to grow too fast."

"Did I cause it?" Mrs. Patel asks.

"No," Leah says firmly. "This isn't a failure or a punishment."

They discuss topical steroids (gl), vitamin D analogs (gl), phototherapy (gl), and screening for joint symptoms. Instructions are printed clearly, without jargon.

12:15 — Lunch, interrupted

Leah manages three bites of lunch before an MA appears.

"Walk-in with a rapidly changing mole."

"Okay," Leah says, standing. "Let's feed pathology first."

The lesion on the young man's back is irregular, dark, and uneven. This one tightens her chest.

She proceeds efficiently: history, dermatoscope, consent, excisional biopsy (gl) with adequate margins.

"This could be benign," she says evenly, "or something we never ignore. Either way, we're acting early."

Only after the specimen is sent does she finish her now-lukewarm lunch.

13:30 — Afternoon rhythm: freezing, reassuring, repeating

Liquid nitrogen for actinic keratoses (gl). Reassurance about scars. Education for molluscum contagiosum (gl). Gentle correction of essential-oil-induced contact dermatitis (gl).

She repeats the same truths all afternoon:

“Benign means not cancer.”

“Patterns over time matter more than a snapshot.”

“Skin tone changes how rashes appear — not how real they are.”

Her sunscreen counseling is practical, never shaming. “I’m not trying to turn you into a vampire,” she jokes. “I want your future self to thank you.”

15:00 — Biologics and cautious hope

Mr. Hernandez has lived with severe plaque psoriasis for years. He is tired of hope.

Leah reviews how biologics target specific immune pathways, discusses infection risks and TB (tuberculosis) (gl) screening, and demonstrates injection technique step by step.

When he practices with the trainer pen, his hands tremble — then steady.

“What if this doesn’t work?” he asks.

“Then we adjust,” Leah says. “But if it does, you may have to remind yourself how bad it used to be.”

16:30 — Post-Mohs reality check

Mrs. Greene examines her sutured nose in the mirror. “I look awful.”

“You look like you’re healing,” Leah says. She explains scar maturation, checks for infection, and outlines scar care with petrolatum (gl), sun protection, and future options.

“What do you want this scar to mean?” Leah asks.

"That I came in when I should have," Mrs. Greene says.

"That's a good story," Leah replies.

17:15 — The add-on that matters

A young woman with a family history of melanoma waits in tears. The mole doesn't scream danger, but it doesn't fully behave either.

"If it worries you," Leah says, "and we can remove it safely, I'd rather let pathology decide."

The biopsy is quick. The relief is visible.

"If it's bad?" the patient asks.

"Then it's small," Leah says. "And small is workable."

18:05 — Closing loops

Leah documents carefully, calls patients with results, flags overdue melanoma follow-ups. Skin cancer does not respect procrastination.

19:00 — Home, mirror, meaning

At home, she showers away the clinic — chlorhexidine (gl), nitrogen, the day. She does a brief self-exam out of habit, noting familiar scars and freckles.

Miguel sets dinner down. "Save any skin today?"

"A few," Leah says. "Caught a maybe. Gave someone hope. Made someone less afraid of their reflection."

Later, she types one line into her notes app:

"Dermatology isn't about perfection. It's about catching dangerous edits early — and helping people feel at home in the skin that carries their life."

Tomorrow will bring new lesions, new fears, new decisions.

Same work: seeing past the spots to the person living inside them.

Chapter 24

Day in the Life — Oncology Nurse Practitioner

(Inpatient Oncology Consult Service 07:00–19:00)

05:50 — Early light, unfinished sleep.

The alarm goes off before the sky commits to morning. It's that thin gray light that feels borrowed, not earned.

Maria sits up slowly, giving her body a moment to catch up. Inpatient consult days feel heavier before they start. There's no infusion schedule to anchor the hours, no predictable arc. Just patients whose cancer has complicated something else — or whose something else has complicated their cancer.

She pulls on scrubs, hair into a low knot, coffee poured but barely tasted. On the counter, a sticky note from last night reads: "Milk. Dog food. Don't forget yourself."

She leaves it where it is.

06:40 — Parking garage math.

The hospital garage smells like concrete and yesterday's rain. Maria parks on level four, where the elevator works most of the time.

As she walks, she opens the consult list on her phone:

- New admission: metastatic colon cancer with bowel obstruction

- Neutropenic fever (gl) overnight in a patient on active chemo

- Known pancreatic cancer, now with new jaundice

- "Goals of care discussion requested" — no other context

Four consults before rounds even begin.

She exhales once. Not dread. Calibration.

07:10 — The consult room that isn't a room.

The oncology workroom is a narrow space with three computers, a printer that jams when you're already late, and a whiteboard listing names that never seem to get erased fast enough.

The fellow is already there, sleeves rolled up, scanning labs.

"Morning," he says. "It's... a day."

Maria smiles. "That's oncology's brand."

They divide the list. She takes the neutropenic fever and the goals-of-care consult first. He'll start with the obstruction.

She logs into Epic (gl), scrolling through overnight vitals, labs, nursing notes. Absolute neutrophil count (ANC) (gl) flagged in red. Blood cultures pending. Broad-spectrum antibiotics already started.

"Good," she murmurs. "Someone didn't wait."

07:45 — Neutropenic fever: quiet urgency.

Room 812 smells faintly of antiseptic and fear.

Mr. Alvarez, 58, lies propped on pillows, skin sallow, eyes alert. His wife sits stiffly in the corner, hands folded too neatly.

"Hi, I'm Maria," she says. "I'm one of the oncology NPs following you while you're here."

"I spiked a fever," he says. "They freaked out."

"They took it seriously," Maria corrects gently. "Which is what we want."

She reviews the plan out loud: cultures, IV antibiotics, fluids, growth factor if counts don't recover. She listens to his lungs, checks his port site, scans the monitor.

"To be clear," she adds, looking at both of them, "this doesn't mean your chemo failed. It means your immune system is doing exactly what we knew it might do."

His wife's shoulders drop an inch.

In the chart, it will read: "Neutropenic fever, stable, continue current management."

In the room, it's reassurance carefully measured so it doesn't drift into false promise.

08:50 — Hallway consults and half conversations.

Between rooms, Maria fields questions:

A nurse asks if a platelet transfusion (gl) threshold should be adjusted.

A resident wants to clarify whether steroids should be held before imaging.

Pharmacy messages about renal dosing on an antibiotic.

Each answer is small. Together, they form the invisible scaffolding holding the day up.

She updates Epic (gl) notes in bursts, saving drafts because someone always knocks before she finishes.

09:30 — Obstruction consult: anatomy and limits.

In room 745, a CT scan glows on the screen. Loops of bowel outlined in stark contrast.

Mr. Peterson, 71, stares at the image like it might explain itself.

The fellow summarizes. Maria watches his face.

“So... surgery?” Mr. Peterson asks.

“Not safely,” Maria says. “Not with where the cancer is.”

She explains decompression, symptom control, possible stenting, what’s realistic and what isn’t. She draws a simple sketch — not to teach anatomy, but to slow the moment down.

“What happens if it doesn’t work?” his daughter asks quietly.

Maria doesn’t rush the answer.

“Then we focus on comfort,” she says. “And on making sure we’re not causing more harm than help.”

There is a long pause. This is not a dramatic conversation. It is a precise one.

10:45 — Jaundice and the waiting game.

The pancreatic cancer patient is young. Too young, everyone thinks, even though cancer doesn't care.

Her bilirubin (gl) is climbing. Eyes yellowed just enough to notice.

Maria reviews imaging, calls GI about ERCP (endoscopic retrograde cholangiopancreatography) (gl) timing, adjusts anti-itch meds. She explains why chemo is on hold for now.

"So we just... wait?" the patient asks.

"We manage what we can," Maria says. "And we don't pretend waiting means doing nothing."

The patient nods, unconvinced but listening.

12:10 — Lunch that barely counts.

Lunch is a protein bar eaten standing up while reviewing labs. Potassium low in one patient. Creatinine creeping in another.

She orders repletion (gl), flags trends, sends messages that will be read later and acted on sooner than anyone realizes.

The pager vibrates twice. She ignores it once. Answers it the second time.

No emergency. Just accumulation.

13:30 — Goals of care: the hard consult.

The chart is thin. The situation is not.

Ms. Reynolds, late 60s, metastatic lung cancer, now intubated after respiratory failure. Family at bedside. The primary team wants oncology "input."

Maria reads between the lines.

She meets the family in a quiet room with bad chairs.

They ask if more chemo would help. They ask if she can "fight harder."

Maria explains prognosis, not in numbers but in trajectories. She explains what treatment can and cannot fix.

"What would you want if this were you?" someone asks.

She answers carefully. "I'd want to be comfortable. And I'd want my family to know they didn't give up on me — they chose me."

There are tears. There is silence. There is relief mixed with grief.

In Epic (gl), she documents: "Discussed goals of care extensively. Family considering comfort-focused approach."

15:10 — The afternoon compression.

Afternoons compress time.

She circles back to earlier consults, adjusts plans, answers pages that stack up while she was in meetings.

One patient's fever resolved. Another's labs worsened. One family wants another conversation.

She calls the outpatient oncologist for continuity, leaves a voicemail that includes both data and nuance.

"Call me," she ends. "There's more to this than the labs."

17:30 — Rounds without ceremony.

The team regroups. Updates exchanged quickly. No one has time for speeches.

They talk thresholds, contingencies, overnight watch points.

Maria writes handoff notes for the night NP: who's fragile, who's anxious, who will call even if nothing changes.

This is not pessimism. It's preparation.

18:45 — Leaving the building.

The hospital is louder at night, oddly. Fewer people, more echoes.

Maria logs out of Epic (gl), shoulders her bag, and pauses at the elevator. Another consult came in ten minutes ago. It can wait until morning.

She steps into the garage, air cool against her face.

Inpatient oncology doesn't offer closure. It offers containment. You hold what you can, pass the rest forward, and trust the system to keep moving.

19:30 — Home, quieter weight.

Dinner is leftovers. The dog leans heavily against her leg.

She answers one last message from a colleague, then sets the phone face down.

Today had no victories. It had prevented disasters. It had softened edges. It had kept people from being alone in moments they didn't choose.

Tomorrow, more consults. Different names. Same work.

Maria pours a glass of water, sits, and lets the day settle — not disappear, just settle enough to sleep.

SCRUB*fits*™ Reflection — Anna Remedy, DNP, FNP-BC, PMHNP

"Across all Nurse Practitioner settings, sustainability is shaped not only by workload, but by how well the daily decision-making rhythm matches how you naturally operate. Pay attention to how the responsibilities described in this chapter feel in your imagination. When people ignore those signals early, burnout often follows later. When they listen to them, career longevity becomes much more achievable."

Chapter 25

The 101™ — The Answers That Decide Long-Term Fit

Most people approach the Nurse Practitioner path looking for answers. Clear ones. Reassuring ones. The kind that reduce uncertainty and confirm that the decision ahead is the right one.

This section is not designed to do that.

The questions that matter most in healthcare careers are rarely the ones with clean, definitive answers. They are the ones that surface tradeoffs, expose assumptions, and force you to confront what you are actually choosing — not just what you hope the role will provide. The 101 questions that follow are not meant to persuade you toward or away from becoming a Nurse Practitioner. They are meant to help you think more accurately about the decision you are making and the life that decision shapes over time.

Many career guides present information as if clarity comes from completeness: lists of duties, scopes of practice, salary ranges, and educational requirements. That information is useful, but it is insufficient. It describes the role from the outside. These questions are concerned with what happens on the inside — inside the workday, inside decision-making, and inside the person carrying responsibility year after year.

The Nurse Practitioner role is often discussed as a destination. In reality, it is a long-term relationship between a person, a system, and a set of expectations that evolve over time. Early enthusiasm, mid-career normalization, and later reassessment are not anomalies; they are common phases. The questions in this section are organized to reflect that arc. Some are most relevant before you apply to school. Others matter most when you are choosing your first role, navigating early practice, or quietly reassessing sustainability years later.

You are not expected to read these questions in order or to answer them all at once. In fact, doing so would miss their purpose. These questions are designed to be returned to at different moments, when context has shifted and your priorities have changed. A question that feels abstract early on may feel urgent later. A question that once felt hypothetical may become concrete after lived experience.

Each answer is intentionally concise. That is not because the issues are simple, but because clarity often comes from restraint rather than exhaustiveness. The goal is not to resolve every uncertainty, but to sharpen your awareness of what you are weighing. If a question lingers with you, that is not a flaw in the answer. It is a signal that the question is doing its job.

You will notice that many of these questions are not about competence. They do not ask whether you are smart enough, capable enough, or resilient enough. Those assumptions dominate much of healthcare education, and they often obscure more important considerations. Being able to do the work is different from being able to live inside it sustainably. These questions are designed to help you explore that difference honestly.

You will also notice that these questions do not treat resume building, job hunting, or interviewing as purely tactical exercises. How you position yourself, how you choose environments, and how you evaluate offers are not administrative details; they are early expressions of alignment. Poor early choices can amplify strain for years. Thoughtful ones can protect growth, safety, and optionality.

This section does not assume that staying is virtuous or that leaving is failure. It does not frame endurance as a moral achievement. It recognizes that healthcare careers unfold within systems that place uneven demands on individuals, and that reassessment is often a rational response rather than a personal shortcoming. The purpose of these questions is not to harden you, but to help you choose with clarity rather than inertia.

Some readers will find confirmation here. Others will find friction. Both outcomes are appropriate. If the questions make the path feel clearer and more grounded, that is information. If they introduce hesitation or discomfort, that is also information. Discomfort does not mean you are on the wrong path. It means you are paying attention.

You are not required to have answers before you move forward. What matters is that you know which questions you are carrying with you — and which ones you are ignoring. The cost of a healthcare career is rarely paid all at once. It is paid over time, through accumulated decisions, expectations, and compromises. The questions that follow are intended to make those costs visible while you still have room to choose.

Use this section as a reference, not a verdict. Return to it when circumstances change. Let different questions matter at different times. The most important outcome is not certainty, but alignment — the ability to make decisions that fit who you are, how you are wired, and what you need to sustain a meaningful life in healthcare.

Becoming & Being a Nurse Practitioner — 100 Questions & Answers

Foundations & Calling (Q1–Q20)

1. What is a Nurse Practitioner (NP)?

A Nurse Practitioner is an advanced practice registered nurse (APRN) who merges hands-on nursing wisdom with the clinical decision-making of a medical provider. NPs diagnose conditions, prescribe medications, and manage treatment plans with an emphasis on holistic, person-centered care. What makes them unique is their ability to combine evidence-based medical practice with the empathy and trust-building traditionally associated with nursing. At their core, NPs are clinicians who don't just treat symptoms — they elevate the entire experience of care.

2. How is an NP different from a registered nurse (RN)?

RNs are the backbone of patient care — they monitor, advocate, and implement treatment plans with exceptional skill. NPs build on that foundation by stepping into roles that involve diagnosing conditions, prescribing medications, and directing care independently or collaboratively. The NP role brings more autonomy, more responsibility, and a broader clinical scope. Together, RNs and NPs form a continuum of care that spans compassion, expertise, and leadership.

3. Why do people choose to become NPs?

Many choose the NP path because they want more influence over patient outcomes while still staying close to the human side of healthcare. They're often driven by a desire to blend critical thinking with meaningful connection. Becoming an NP allows someone to shape care with both authority and empathy, offering solutions that honor the whole person. For many, the decision feels less like a career move and more like answering a calling.

4. Is the NP path right for everyone?

No single healthcare role fits every personality, even one as impactful as this. The NP journey is best suited for people who embrace responsibility, uncertainty, and lifelong learning. It requires a unique mix of resilience, curiosity, and compassion. Alignment — who you are and what the role demands — determines long-term success far more than ambition alone.

5. What's the biggest misconception about NPs?

A common misconception is that NPs are "almost doctors," which oversimplifies and misrepresents the profession. Nurse Practitioners are not defined by comparison — they're a distinct role rooted in nursing philosophy and holistic care. Their strength lies in blending clinical expertise with patient partnership, not in mimicking anyone else. When people understand this, they begin to appreciate NPs for what they truly are: independent, evidence-informed healers.

6. Are NPs in demand?

Absolutely — the profession is expanding faster than almost any other healthcare role in the country. The growth is fueled by physician shortages, aging populations, chronic disease, and the shift toward team-based care. Communities rely on NPs to increase access, decrease wait times, and provide high-quality primary and specialty services. The demand is expected to rise steadily for years to come.

7. What values define a great NP?

Great NPs are anchored in empathy — the ability to listen without judgment and respond with humanity. They uphold integrity and accountability, recognizing that each decision affects a person's life. Curiosity drives them to keep learning, questioning, and improving. And courage allows them to advocate boldly, even when the path is difficult or unpopular.

8. What's the most rewarding part of being an NP?

The most rewarding moments often happen quietly: a patient finally breathing easier, a family feeling heard, or a child trusting you enough to smile during an exam. NPs see progress in real time and get to witness healing unfold. They also build relationships that extend well beyond a single visit, creating continuity and genuine connection. Knowing you helped guide someone toward better health is a reward that never fades.

9. What's the hardest part?

Time pressure is an ever-present challenge — appointments are short, documentation is long, and needs are endless. Emotional fatigue can build, especially when caring for patients in crisis or managing chronic illness with limited resources. The complexity of modern healthcare demands constant juggling of priorities. Yet with strong boundaries and support, many NPs turn these challenges into sources of strength.

10. What kinds of patients do NPs see?

NPs treat a stunning variety of individuals across the lifespan. Depending on their specialty, they may care for newborns, teenagers, athletes, pregnant patients, older adults, or people navigating chronic conditions. Every day brings new stories, new challenges, and new opportunities to impact someone's life. The diversity keeps the work meaningful and dynamic.

11. Can NPs specialize?

Yes — specialization is one of the strengths of the NP profession. Whether someone is drawn to pediatrics, mental health, acute care, women's health, geriatrics, or family practice, there's a path that matches their passion. Specializing allows NPs to develop deep expertise in a focused area of medicine. It's a way to align interests, talents, and long-term career goals.

12. How do NPs impact healthcare access?

NPs are essential in communities where medical providers are scarce. They reduce wait times, expand clinic hours, and often serve as the primary care provider for underserved populations. By bringing care to rural towns, community clinics, and low-access neighborhoods, they close gaps that would otherwise leave people without help. Their presence doesn't just improve access — it improves outcomes.

13. How do NPs embody alignment?

Alignment for an NP means practicing in a way that honors both their clinical training and their human values. It's the harmony between purpose, passion, and professional responsibilities. An aligned NP feels grounded, energized, and deeply connected to their work. When that alignment is present, both the patient and the clinician thrive.

14. Who supervises NPs?

Supervision varies based on state laws and facility policies. In full practice authority states, NPs practice independently without mandatory physician oversight. In other regions, they collaborate with physicians while still maintaining a high level of autonomy. Regardless of the structure, NPs are recognized as advanced, highly skilled clinicians who lead patient care.

15. What's full practice authority (FPA)?

Full practice authority means NPs can evaluate, diagnose, and treat patients — including prescribing medications — without physician supervision. This model is endorsed by major healthcare organizations because it improves access and maintains high-quality outcomes. Over half of U.S. states have implemented FPA, and the momentum continues to grow. For NPs, FPA represents both professional empowerment and expanded community impact.

16. Can NPs open their own clinics?

Yes, NPs can open independent clinics in states with full practice authority. Many operate successful practices in primary care, women's health, aesthetics, and wellness services. Owning a clinic offers NPs the chance to design the type of care environment they believe patients deserve. It also allows them to innovate, lead, and create sustainable community health models.

17. What type of personality fits this role?

The NP role is best suited for individuals who blend analytical thinking with emotional intelligence. They must be decisive but also humble enough to collaborate and consult when needed. Curiosity helps them stay sharp, while compassion helps them stay grounded. The most successful NPs are those who can handle complexity while maintaining humanity.

18. How long does it take to become an NP?

From nursing school through NP licensure, the journey typically takes six to eight years. This timeline includes earning a BSN, gaining RN experience, and completing a graduate-level NP program. Some accelerate the process; others stretch it to accommodate work or family life. The path is demanding but deeply rewarding for those who feel called to it.

19. Do all NPs have doctorates?

Not yet — many practicing NPs hold a Master of Science in Nursing (MSN). However, the Doctor of Nursing Practice (DNP) is becoming increasingly common, especially for leadership or system-level roles. The DNP emphasizes quality improvement, healthcare policy, and advanced clinical expertise. Whether MSN or DNP, both pathways produce highly capable clinicians.

20. What's the "color" of Nurse Practitioners in *What Color Are Your Scrubs?* terms?

Nurse Practitioners are represented by **Royal Blue**, a color that embodies calm authority and clinical depth. Royal Blue signals steadiness — the kind of presence that reassures patients even in uncertainty. It also reflects a human-centered approach that balances science with compassion. In the **SCRUB*fit*™** universe, Royal Blue is the shade of trustworthy expertise.

Education & Training (Q21–Q40)

21. What degree do I need to become an NP?

To become an NP, you'll need either a Master of Science in Nursing (MSN) or a Doctor of Nursing Practice (DNP) from an accredited program. Both pathways prepare you with advanced clinical knowledge, but the DNP adds training in leadership, policy, and population health. Think of the MSN as the minimum entry point and the DNP as the long-term evolution of the profession. No matter which degree you choose, what matters most is that the program is aligned with your specialty and fully prepares you for real-world practice.

22. What are the common NP specialties?

The most common specialties include Family Nurse Practitioner (FNP), Adult-Gerontology (AGNP), Pediatric (PNP), Women's Health (WHNP), Acute Care (ACNP), and Psych-Mental Health (PMHNP). Each specialty carries its own rhythm, clinical focus, and patient population. For example, FNPs see patients across the lifespan, while PMHNPs dive deeply into mental and behavioral health. The variety allows future NPs to choose a path that matches their natural strengths and the communities they want to serve.

23. How do I choose a specialty?

Choosing a specialty should feel like matching your heartbeat to your future clinical home. Start by reflecting on the populations and environments where you feel most energized — pediatrics, mental health, acute care, or primary care. Think about the pace you enjoy, the stories that move you, and the problems you feel called to solve. Your specialty should feel less like a decision and more like recognition: *This is where I belong.*

24. Is it better to work as an RN first?

Yes — RN experience is a powerful foundation for NP practice, even if not always required. Those years at the bedside teach communication, prioritization, patient advocacy, and the subtle art of clinical judgment. When you step into the NP role, those instincts carry forward and guide your decision-making. While some pathways allow direct progression, real-world experience often becomes an invaluable asset later.

25. How long is NP school?

Most MSN programs take 2–3 years to complete, depending on whether you enroll full-time or part-time. DNP programs usually take 3–4 years, especially if you're adding a capstone or clinical scholarship project. Many programs are now hybrid or flexible to support working nurses. The timeline is rigorous, but the transformation that occurs along the way is worth every late night and clinical hour.

26. What are clinical hours?

Clinical hours are hands-on training experiences where you work with real patients under the guidance of NP or physician preceptors. They typically range between 500 and 1,000 hours, depending on program and specialty. These hours bridge the gap between theory and practice, allowing you to apply classroom learning in real-world scenarios. They're the moments where you discover your strengths, refine your voice, and grow into your new role.

27. How do I find a preceptor?

Finding a preceptor can take time and strategic outreach. Start early by connecting with clinics, hospitals, alumni networks, and local NP associations. Many students also secure preceptors through colleagues, mentors, or by building relationships during their RN practice. Persistence and professionalism go a long way — the right preceptor can shape your confidence and clinical style for years to come.

28. Are NP programs hard?

Yes — NP programs are challenging, but in a purposeful, growth-oriented way. You'll study advanced pathophysiology, pharmacology, diagnostics, and clinical reasoning. The workload demands discipline, but it also builds pride and resilience. If you're driven by purpose and willing to put in the effort, the difficulty becomes part of the reward.

29. What's the difference between MSN and DNP?

The MSN prepares you for entry-level NP practice, equipping you with the knowledge and clinical hours needed to care for patients at an advanced level. The DNP goes further by adding leadership, systems thinking, and population health training. Many who pursue the DNP do so to influence healthcare policy, lead quality improvement projects, or stabilize long-term career growth. Both are respected — the choice depends on your vision for your future.

30. Are online NP programs respected?

Accredited online programs are widely respected, especially when paired with strong clinical experiences. Employers care less about the format and more about the competencies you demonstrate. Online learning can be a lifeline for working nurses balancing shifts, family, and school. What matters most is your commitment, your training, and the quality of the program you choose.

31. Can you work during NP school?

Yes, many students work part-time or even full-time during NP school, especially in the early semesters. However, balancing work with clinical hours and academic demands requires serious time management. Some employers offer flexible scheduling or tuition support, which can make a big difference. Know your limits, stay organized, and give yourself permission to rest when needed.

32. What's the cost of NP education?

MSN programs typically range from $35,000 to $70,000, depending on the school and location. DNP programs may range from $60,000 to $120,000, especially at larger universities. While these numbers can feel intimidating, many students offset costs through financial aid, employer tuition reimbursement, and scholarships. Think of it as a long-term investment in a career with stability, flexibility, and impact.

33. How can I fund NP school?

There are several options: scholarships, federal student aid, HRSA loan forgiveness programs, and employer tuition reimbursement. Some organizations offer funding specifically for nurses working in underserved areas. Military service and public health commitments can also reduce educational costs dramatically. Don't overlook smaller scholarships — they add up faster than you think.

34. What's NP certification?

After completing your degree, you must take a national board certification exam through AANP or ANCC, depending on your specialty. Certification validates your knowledge and allows you to practice legally as an NP. Most students study for months using review courses, practice exams, and question banks. Passing boards is a moment of realization — you've earned your place in the profession.

35. Do I need a license in every state?

Yes, you must hold an NP license in each state where you practice. Many states are moving toward the APRN Compact, which will allow NPs to hold a multi-state license similar to RNs. Until then, licensing remains state-specific, and requirements may vary. It's wise to familiarize yourself with local regulations early, especially if you plan to move or practice telehealth.

36. Are there bridge programs?

Yes — bridge programs such as RN-to-MSN and BSN-to-DNP pathways streamline the journey for nurses entering advanced practice. These programs are designed to honor prior experience while accelerating academic progression. They're ideal for motivated nurses who want to become NPs without unnecessary delays. Bridge programs make the profession more accessible to a diverse range of learners and career backgrounds.

37. What's the best way to prepare for NP boards?

The best preparation is consistent, focused study combined with high-quality question banks. Start early and review a little each day rather than cramming. Many students benefit from live or online review courses that reinforce clinical judgment and exam strategy. Treat studying as training — every question strengthens your readiness.

38. Can NPs subspecialize?

Yes — many NPs pursue additional training in cardiology, oncology, dermatology, endocrinology, nephrology, or other specialized fields. These post-graduate certificates deepen your expertise and open new career doors. Subspecialization is especially helpful for NPs who enjoy complex cases or want to work in high-acuity settings. Your career can evolve with your curiosity — and that's one of the profession's greatest strengths.

39. What's the hardest part of NP school?

Time management is often the biggest challenge — juggling clinical hours, classes, family, and work simultaneously. The academic load can feel heavy, especially during semesters with pharmacology or pathophysiology. Many students struggle with imposter syndrome, wondering if they're truly ready for advanced practice. But growth happens under pressure, and most look back amazed at what they accomplished.

40. How do you stay motivated?

Motivation grows when you stay connected to your "why" — the reason you chose this path in the first place. Write it down, say it out loud, or keep it somewhere you see daily. Supportive classmates, mentors, and family members can reignite your confidence on tough days. Every step forward, no matter how small, is proof that you're becoming the clinician you once hoped to be.

Clinical Practice & Scope (Q41–Q60)

41. What's a typical NP workday like?

A typical NP workday blends clinical focus with human connection. You might move between patient visits, charting, reviewing labs, coordinating care, and collaborating with your team. Each encounter requires a shift in mindset — from acute concerns to chronic management to preventive guidance. Every day carries its own rhythm, but the constant is this: you're balancing science with storytelling, facts with feelings, and data with lived experience.

42. How many patients do NPs see daily?

The number varies widely based on specialty, setting, and patient complexity. Primary care NPs may see 15–25 patients in a day, while acute care or specialty NPs may see fewer but more complex cases. The goal isn't volume — it's quality, safety, and connection. Great NPs adapt their pace to the needs of the moment while keeping care centered on the patient, not the clock.

43. Do NPs prescribe medications?

Yes, NPs can prescribe medications in every state, including controlled substances in most regions. Prescribing isn't just about selecting a drug — it involves weighing risks, benefits, interactions, and patient preferences. NPs also prioritize nonpharmacologic interventions when appropriate, in line with holistic nursing philosophy. This combination of clinical judgment and patient partnership defines NP prescribing.

44. Can NPs admit patients to hospitals?

In many states and health systems, NPs can admit patients, especially if they hold hospital privileges. This ability allows them to follow patients across the continuum of care, strengthening relationships and ensuring continuity. Hospital policies may vary, but NPs increasingly function as essential members of inpatient teams. Their role bridges outpatient insight with inpatient needs, improving safety and outcomes.

45. What's the role of evidence-based practice?

Evidence-based practice is the backbone of NP decision-making. It means integrating the best available research with clinical expertise and the patient's unique values and circumstances. This approach keeps care current, safe, and effective. NPs are trained to evaluate studies, challenge outdated practices, and advocate for solutions grounded in science.

46. Do NPs perform procedures?

Yes — NPs perform a wide range of procedures depending on their specialty and training. This might include suturing, I&Ds, biopsies, pap smears, IUD insertions, joint injections, or even advanced procedures in acute settings. Procedures allow NPs to deliver efficient, comprehensive care in real time. The skill is not just technical; it includes patient coaching, consent, comfort, and follow-up.

47. How much autonomy do NPs have?

Autonomy varies greatly by state and facility, but the trend is toward increasing independence. In full-practice states, NPs can diagnose, treat, and prescribe without physician oversight. In collaborative states, autonomy remains high but may require formal agreements. Regardless of location, NPs are respected as advanced clinicians capable of leading care with confidence and accountability.

48. How do NPs collaborate with physicians?

NPs collaborate as colleagues, not subordinates. They share information, consult on complex cases, and align on treatment plans when interdisciplinary insight enhances outcomes. Collaboration is rooted in mutual respect and shared commitment to patient care. The dynamic looks different in every environment, but at its best, it reflects teamwork without hierarchy.

49. What documentation systems do NPs use?

NPs primarily use Electronic Health Records (EHRs) such as Epic, Cerner, Meditech, or Athena. Documentation captures clinical findings, supports billing, and ensures continuity across providers. While EHRs can feel time-consuming, mastery of templates, smart phrases, and workflows can dramatically improve efficiency. Good documentation isn't just a task — it's a safeguard for patients and clinicians alike.

50. How do NPs handle emergencies?

NPs approach emergencies with calm, clarity, and swift clinical reasoning. They stabilize the patient, initiate protocols, and call for additional support when needed. Training in rapid assessment allows them to make crucial decisions under pressure. While emergencies are intense, they also highlight the strength, skill, and steadiness of NP practice.

51. What's the difference between acute and primary care NPs?

Acute care NPs focus on unstable or complex conditions in settings like ICUs, emergency departments, and inpatient units. Primary care NPs specialize in prevention, chronic disease management, and long-term relationships with patients. The distinction lies less in ability and more in the population's acuity and needs. Both paths require advanced knowledge, but each calls to a different type of clinician.

52. How do NPs manage chronic conditions?

NPs blend medical treatment with lifestyle coaching, education, and long-term monitoring. They help patients understand their conditions and empower them to take ownership of their health. This partnership approach makes chronic disease feel less overwhelming and more manageable. Over time, NPs become trusted guides who celebrate small wins and help navigate inevitable setbacks.

53. What role does patient education play?

Patient education is central to NP care — it's where understanding transforms into action. NPs translate complex medical information into everyday language, giving patients the power to make informed choices. Education builds confidence, reduces fear, and strengthens partnership. When patients understand the "why" behind a plan, outcomes almost always improve.

54. Do NPs make house calls?

Yes, some NPs provide home-based care, especially in palliative, geriatric, concierge, or home health settings. House calls allow NPs to see patients in their real environments, revealing context that clinics often miss. This kind of care builds trust and reduces barriers for patients who cannot travel. It's a return to medicine's roots — bringing care directly to the person.

55. Can NPs work internationally?

Yes, though licensing and scope vary by country. Many NPs participate in global health initiatives, humanitarian aid, or medical missions. International work offers perspective, cultural humility, and a renewed appreciation for resourceful, adaptable care. NPs who enjoy adventure and service often find global work deeply transforming.

56. What's the NP's role in mental health?

Psych-Mental Health NPs (PMHNPs) diagnose and treat psychiatric disorders, manage medications, and provide therapeutic support. Even non-PMHNPs play an essential role in recognizing early symptoms, screening patients, and initiating referrals. Mental health touches every part of healthcare, making NPs crucial in destigmatizing conversations and expanding access. Their holistic approach is especially powerful in addressing both mind and body.

57. How do NPs prevent burnout?

Preventing burnout requires intentional boundaries, self-reflection, and a commitment to sustainable practice. NPs must honor their limits, take breaks, and cultivate supportive relationships both inside and outside the clinic. Alignment plays a huge role — being in the wrong environment drains faster than any long shift. When NPs care for themselves as fiercely as they care for others, longevity becomes possible.

58. How do NPs use technology?

NPs use telehealth, EHRs, mobile diagnostics, wearable data, and digital communication tools to extend care beyond traditional walls. Technology enhances efficiency and accessibility, especially for patients with mobility or transportation barriers. It also allows NPs to track long-term data trends that improve clinical decision-making. When used thoughtfully, technology strengthens the NP-patient connection rather than replacing it.

59. Are NPs respected by other clinicians?

Yes — respect grows naturally when NPs demonstrate competence, professionalism, and collaboration. Physicians, nurses, and allied health professionals increasingly recognize NPs as vital contributors to patient care. Respect is rarely automatic; it is earned through consistency and evidence-based practice. Over time, NPs become trusted partners in the shared mission of improving health.

60. How do patients view NPs?

Patients often describe NPs as approachable, relatable clinicians who blend medical expertise with genuine empathy. They appreciate the time NPs spend explaining diagnoses, listening to concerns, and involving them in decisions. Many patients feel more comfortable opening up to NPs, which strengthens trust and improves outcomes. In countless clinics across the country, patients say the same thing: “My NP really listens to me.”

Career Growth & Leadership (Q61–Q80)

61. What leadership roles can NPs pursue?

NPs can rise into leadership roles such as clinical directors, practice managers, department chiefs, and advanced practice supervisors. Their experience at the bedside gives them a unique perspective on patient needs and system flaws, which strengthens their leadership voice. Many NPs also serve as policy advisors, consultants, or founders of innovative care models. Leadership isn't a separate path for NPs — it's a natural expansion of their impact.

62. Do NPs teach?

Yes — many NPs teach in universities, residency programs, and hospitals. Teaching allows NPs to shape the next generation of clinicians and share the wisdom gained from real-world practice. Whether leading a classroom, precepting students, or mentoring peers, teaching is a form of legacy-building. It's a way to magnify your influence far beyond your own patient panel.

63. What's the DNP's advantage in leadership?

The Doctor of Nursing Practice (DNP) equips NPs to influence systems, not just individual patient cases. It focuses on quality improvement, healthcare policy, leadership, and change management — the levers that shape entire organizations. DNP-prepared NPs often lead initiatives that reduce errors, improve patient satisfaction, and transform workflows. The degree adds depth and credibility, helping NPs sit at decision-making tables where their voices matter most.

64. How can NPs advocate for patients?

Advocacy begins with listening — truly understanding what a patient needs, fears, or hopes for. NPs advocate through education, by explaining conditions in ways that empower rather than overwhelm. They also advocate at system levels: pushing for policy changes, safety improvements, and equitable access. Every time an NP speaks up for a patient, they strengthen trust and humanize healthcare.

65. What's the salary range for NPs?

Most NPs earn between $120K and $160K annually, though salaries vary by specialty, region, and experience. High-demand fields like psychiatric, neonatal, and acute care tend to offer higher compensation. Beyond salary, many NPs appreciate benefits such as flexible scheduling, loan repayment programs, and robust clinical autonomy. Compensation reflects not just what NPs do — but the depth and breadth of their impact.

66. Which specialties earn the most?

Psychiatric-Mental Health, Neonatal, and Acute Care NPs typically earn the highest salaries due to demand and intensity of practice. These specialties require advanced expertise, high responsibility, and comfort managing complex conditions. Compensation increases with experience, certifications, and leadership roles. Ultimately, the "best" specialty is the one where passion and purpose intersect.

67. What's the job outlook?

The job outlook for NPs is exceptionally strong, with consistent growth across all states. Demand is fueled by physician shortages, aging populations, chronic disease, and the shift to value-based care. NPs are increasingly recognized as essential to modern healthcare's sustainability and accessibility. The profession's future is not just bright — it's expanding.

68. How can NPs grow professionally?

Professional growth happens through lifelong learning. NPs can join professional associations, attend conferences, publish research, or present at clinical meetings. Many expand their impact by precepting students, obtaining additional certifications, or pursuing fellowships. Growth isn't a single path — it's the decision to keep evolving in pursuit of better care.

69. Are NPs part of unions?

In some regions and hospital systems, NPs join unions to advocate for safe staffing, fair compensation, and improved working conditions. Union membership gives NPs a collective voice in negotiations that shape their day-to-day practice. Not all states or employers offer union options, but where available, they can be powerful tools for change. Whether unionized or not, NPs remain strong advocates for professional protections.

70. How do NPs gain leadership credibility?

Credibility comes from consistency — showing up prepared, informed, and centered every day. NPs earn trust by delivering evidence-based care, communicating clearly, and remaining accountable under pressure. Their actions, more than their titles, prove their readiness to lead. When clinicians demonstrate both competence and compassion, credibility grows naturally.

71. Can NPs run hospitals or clinics?

Yes — NPs can lead clinics, departments, and even entire healthcare organizations. Leadership roles such as CEO, chief nursing officer, or clinical director are increasingly filled by advanced practice clinicians. Their blend of administrative insight and clinical experience makes them well-suited for guiding modern healthcare systems. Running a clinic or hospital isn't just possible for NPs — many are already doing it.

72. What's the difference between leadership and management?

Management focuses on processes, scheduling, organization, and operational flow. Leadership, on the other hand, inspires people, shapes vision, and builds culture. NPs often find themselves doing both, especially in team-based environments. The most effective NPs know when to manage and when to lead — balancing structure with inspiration.

73. Can NPs work in research?

Absolutely — NPs play a vital role in clinical research, quality improvement studies, and evidence generation. They bring firsthand patient experience to research questions that matter in real-world practice. NPs may serve as principal investigators, research coordinators, or collaborators in multi-disciplinary studies. Research allows NPs to push the profession forward and ensure practice evolves with science.

74. What's professional alignment?

Professional alignment happens when your strengths, values, and role intersect in a way that feels natural and energizing.

An aligned NP feels purposeful, connected, and supported by their environment. Misalignment, by contrast, breeds frustration and exhaustion even in otherwise "good" jobs. Alignment doesn't just improve job satisfaction — it improves longevity and emotional wellbeing.

75. How do NPs use CARESET™?

Nurse Practitioners use **CARESET™** as a practical alignment lens — not a philosophy and not a checklist — to evaluate whether a role, setting, or organization will support sustainable practice.

- **Culture** — Does the clinical culture respect nursing judgment, collaboration, and patient-centered care, or does it undermine professional voice?

- **Autonomy** — Is the NP trusted to practice at the top of licensure with appropriate decision-making authority?

- **Resources** — Are staffing, support systems, technology, and clinical backup sufficient to provide safe, effective care?

- **Expectations** — Are productivity, documentation, call, and availability expectations realistic and transparent?

- **Structure** — Does the workflow, scheduling model, and leadership structure support quality care rather than constant urgency?

- **Environment** — Is the physical and emotional environment conducive to focus, safety, and recovery between demands?

- **Team** — Are interdisciplinary relationships respectful, communicative, and aligned around patient outcomes?

When CARESET™ elements are aligned, Nurse Practitioners feel grounded, effective, and resilient. When one or more elements are misaligned, burnout is rarely a mystery — it is structural, predictable, and preventable.

CARESET™ helps NPs evaluate roles **before committing**, diagnose misalignment **when strain appears**, and make informed pivots **without self-blame**.

76. How can NPs mentor others?

NPs mentor by sharing stories, offering honest advice, and creating space for questions without judgment. Mentorship doesn't require a title — just a willingness to lift others up. Great mentors model resilience, humility, and curiosity. When NPs mentor students or peers, they shape the future of the profession one conversation at a time.

77. What's the connection between Magnet® hospitals and NPs?

Magnet® hospitals are recognized for nursing excellence, evidence-based practice, and strong clinical outcomes. These environments naturally support NPs, who thrive in settings that value nursing leadership and innovation. Magnet organizations invest in advanced education, strong preceptor programs, and collaborative care models. For NPs, working in a Magnet hospital often means greater support, autonomy, and growth opportunities.

78. Can NPs serve in the military?

Yes — NPs serve in all branches of the U.S. military, providing advanced care to service members, veterans, and military families. These roles can include primary care, trauma care, emergency medicine, or specialty services depending on training. Military NPs often develop exceptional skills in adaptability, leadership, and crisis response. Serving as an NP in the military is both an honor and a testament to the profession's versatility.

79. Do NPs write books or conduct media outreach?

Many do — NPs write books, create podcasts, develop educational platforms, and speak on national stages. Their expertise makes them valuable voices in public health communication. Media outreach allows NPs to correct misinformation, promote wellness, and advocate for their profession. The NP voice is increasingly visible, influential, and trusted in healthcare conversations.

80. What legacy can an NP leave?

An NP's legacy lives in the healthier lives they helped shape — the child who grew strong, the adult who managed a chronic condition successfully, the elder who felt respected and cared for. It also lives in the students they mentored and the colleagues they inspired. Legacy isn't measured in years worked, but in lives touched. At their best, NPs leave behind a culture of empathy, advocacy, and clinical excellence.

Real Talk & Reflection (Q81–Q100)

81. What's your best advice for future NPs?

Stay curious — curiosity is the flame that keeps your clinical mind alive. Stay kind — kindness creates trust faster than any prescription. Stay aligned — the work feels lighter when your environment matches your values. And above all, remember that every skill can be learned, but your heart is already enough.

82. What's the biggest early-career mistake?

Overcommitting is the most common early-career trap — saying yes to extra shifts, extra responsibilities, or roles that stretch you too thin. New NPs often feel pressure to prove themselves, but burnout happens quietly and quickly. Growth requires space, boundaries, and honesty about your capacity. The strongest clinicians are the ones who pace themselves intentionally.

83. How do you build confidence?

Confidence grows from preparation, practice, and compassionate self-talk. Every time you make a thoughtful decision, handle a difficult conversation, or ask for help, you expand your competence. Mentors can accelerate this growth by offering guidance and perspective. With time, the moments that once made your heart race become the ones you handle with steady hands.

84. What's one myth about NP school?

A major myth is that you must know exactly what specialty or population you want before you begin. In reality, exposure during school helps reveal your natural strengths and passions. Many NPs discover their calling unexpectedly — in a rotation, a conversation, or a clinical moment that just feels right. Growth is a process, not a prerequisite.

85. How can family support an NP student?

Family can support by offering patience, understanding, and flexibility with time. NP school requires long study hours and emotional bandwidth that may fluctuate. Small gestures — a meal, a quiet space, a simple check-in — can make an enormous difference. When family participates in the journey, the student feels less alone.

86. What's one book every NP should read?

From Silence to Voice: What Nurses Know and Must Communicate to the Public is essential reading for every NP. It teaches clinicians how to articulate their expertise clearly and confidently. The book helps nurses understand that their voice is not optional — it is vital. By learning to speak up, NPs strengthen both their profession and their patients.

87. What's one skill every NP should master?

Active listening is the skill that elevates care from transactional to transformational. When patients feel heard, they reveal details that can change diagnoses and improve outcomes. Listening creates safety, builds trust, and strengthens the therapeutic alliance. It's not just a communication skill — it's a clinical tool.

88. How do NPs manage imposter syndrome?

Managing imposter syndrome begins with acknowledging that almost every clinician feels it at some point. Remind yourself that mastery is earned through practice, not perfection. Seek feedback from mentors and celebrate your progress instead of focusing solely on gaps. Over time, experience transforms doubt into confidence.

89. How can NPs find mentors?

Mentors can be found through professional associations, co-workers, conferences, or preceptor relationships. The key is to approach people with curiosity, humility, and gratitude. Most experienced NPs enjoy helping others succeed — you just have to ask. A good mentor provides guidance, affirmation, and the occasional gentle push forward.

90. What keeps NPs inspired?

Inspiration often comes from small moments: a patient's relief, a successful plan, or a heartfelt "thank you." NPs also draw inspiration from colleagues who show resilience and from students who bring fresh energy. Growth, creativity, and connection keep the work meaningful even during difficult weeks. The profession is demanding, but it is also extraordinarily rewarding.

91. How do NPs handle errors?

NPs address errors with honesty, humility, and a commitment to learning. They follow established safety protocols, communicate transparently with their team, and reflect on what could prevent similar issues in the future. Mistakes are emotionally heavy, but they can be powerful teachers. Owning them builds trust with both patients and colleagues.

92. What's one habit of highly aligned NPs?

Highly aligned NPs practice regular reflection — journaling, debriefing, or simply checking in with themselves. They ask: "What energized me today? What drained me? What does this tell me?" Reflection turns daily experiences into long-term wisdom. It keeps clinicians grounded, intentional, and connected to purpose.

93. How do NPs manage work-life balance?

Balance starts with boundaries — the willingness to say no, delegate, and protect personal time. Humor and connection help offset stress during difficult shifts. Community, whether family, colleagues, or friends, provides emotional fuel. When NPs invest in their own well-being, they show up stronger for others.

94. What's one thing schools don't teach?

Schools rarely teach emotional endurance — the ability to remain present, compassionate, and effective even when you're tired or overwhelmed. This skill is learned on the job, through experience and support. Emotional endurance grows when clinicians practice self-care and lean on their teams. It's the quiet strength that keeps NPs steady year after year.

95. What does success feel like as an NP?

Success rarely feels like fireworks — it often feels like calm. It's the moment when a patient smiles with relief, a plan comes together, or you realize you handled a difficult case with confidence. Success feels like peace: knowing you made a difference that day. Over time, it becomes a quiet, steady sense of purpose.

96. What's one sign you're misaligned in your NP role?

A major sign of misalignment is waking up with consistent dread, even when nothing dramatic has happened at work. Misalignment drains energy faster than any workload. You may feel disconnected from your team, your pace, or your patient population. When these feelings persist, it's time to explore whether a different specialty or setting fits better.

97. Can NPs change specialties later?

Yes — many NPs transition into new specialties through post-graduate certificates or on-the-job training. Healthcare is dynamic, and NPs evolve right along with it. Switching specialties allows clinicians to rediscover passion, pursue new challenges, or align with changing life stages. Your NP career is not a single fixed lane — it's a lifelong journey with many on-ramps.

98. How can NPs give back?

NPs can give back by volunteering in free clinics, participating in community health events, or offering mentorship to students. Teaching, advocacy, and policy involvement are powerful ways to elevate the profession. Giving back keeps clinicians grounded in purpose and connected to the heart of their work. Every contribution, big or small, helps build a healthier, more equitable future.

99. What's the role of gratitude in this work?

Gratitude reframes the difficult moments and highlights the meaningful ones. It reminds NPs why they chose this path and helps prevent emotional fatigue. Gratitude can be directed toward patients, colleagues, mentors, or even oneself. When practiced regularly, it becomes a quiet superpower that sustains resilience.

100. If you could tell your younger self one thing before becoming an NP, what would it be?

"Trust your calling — it knows where you're headed even when you don't."

Your future self would remind you that the science will come, the skills will strengthen, and the confidence will grow. The heart you start with is already the heart patients will need. Every challenge will shape you into the clinician you were meant to become.

101. If I'm being completely honest with myself, should I become a Nurse Practitioner — or would another path fit me better?

This question is not about capability; it is about fit over time. The Nurse Practitioner role demands sustained responsibility, tolerance for uncertainty, and ongoing decision ownership. Some people find that demand clarifying and meaningful across decades. Others find it quietly depleting despite competence and dedication. The honest answer is the one that allows you to build a career you can sustain without losing yourself.

Chapter 26

Find Your Fit, Before You Commit

This is the point in the book where reflection turns into action.

Up to now, the focus has been on understanding the lived reality of the Nurse Practitioner role—what it costs, how it feels, and the kinds of questions that actually determine long-term fit. The sections you've already read are meant to slow you down, not to stall you. They exist to ensure that any next step you take is grounded in clarity rather than momentum.

Find Your Fit, Before You Commit is the bridge between insight and execution.

Healthcare careers have a way of pulling people forward through accumulation: prerequisites lead to applications, applications lead to acceptance, acceptance leads to debt, and debt leads to commitment. At no point in that chain are you explicitly asked to pause and examine whether the role you are moving toward aligns with how you think, decide, recover, and carry responsibility over time. Capability is assumed. Fit is rarely examined.

This framework exists to correct that imbalance.

The purpose of this section is not to persuade you toward or away from becoming a Nurse Practitioner. It is to give you a structured way to test alignment before decisions become difficult—or expensive—to undo. What follows is a practical system designed to be used at multiple moments: before applying to school, while preparing to enter the job market, during interviews and negotiations, and again in the early months of practice.

You can move through these components sequentially, or you can return to them selectively as your circumstances change. The system is designed to support real decision-making, not linear reading.

How This Framework Works

The sections that follow are organized to mirror the actual arc of a healthcare career decision, not the idealized version most people are shown.

You will begin by translating your experience into language that employers understand, without distorting who you are or overselling what the role demands. You will then learn how to locate opportunities that align with your priorities, apply strategically in systems that often filter out strong candidates, and prepare for interviews that assess judgment rather than knowledge.

From there, the focus shifts to negotiation—not as a performance, but as an act of boundary-setting—and finally to the first ninety days of practice, when early misalignment often reveals itself most clearly.

Each component of the framework answers a different question:

- How do I present myself honestly at this stage of my career?
- Where should I actually be looking for roles—and why?
- How do hiring systems work, and how do I navigate them without disappearing?
- What are interviewers really assessing?
- What am I agreeing to when I say yes to an offer?
- How do I stabilize myself in the role before doubt or exhaustion sets in?

Taken together, these sections form a decision system rather than a checklist.

What This Framework Is (and Isn't)

This framework is not about optimization. It will not teach you how to extract the highest possible salary, secure the most prestigious title, or accelerate your trajectory at any cost. Those outcomes may occur, but they are not the goal.

The goal is sustainability.

Fit is not a personality test result or a moment of certainty. It is the ongoing alignment between the demands of a role and the way you function as a human being. When that alignment is close enough, the work remains viable even when it is difficult. When it is not, no amount of competence or external validation will prevent erosion over time.

This framework assumes that you are intelligent, capable, and already motivated. It does not assume that you should tolerate misalignment simply because you *can*.

Using This Section Over Time

You do not need to complete this framework all at once.

Some readers will use it before applying to Nurse Practitioner programs. Others will return to it while job searching, negotiating offers, or reassessing fit after their first year in practice. You may move back and forth between sections as your understanding deepens or as your circumstances change.

That is expected.

The most important thing to remember is that commitment in healthcare often becomes heavier with time, not lighter. Decisions that feel manageable early can become constraining later if they were made without a clear understanding of tradeoffs.

This framework is here to give you that understanding before the stakes rise.

What Comes Next

The sections that follow move deliberately from preparation to execution:

You will begin with **SCRUBScript™**, which addresses how your experience should evolve on paper as your career progresses. From there, **CareerNav™** will help you identify where aligned roles actually exist and how people really get hired. **ApplySmart™** addresses the systems that stand between you and a human reader. **Intelligent Interviews™**

reframes interviews as assessments of judgment and fit rather than performance.

Terms of Care™ will guide you through negotiation as a matter of boundaries and sustainability, not leverage alone. **The 90-Day Pathway™** focuses on early stabilization, when many clinicians discover too late that something is off.

None of these sections exist in isolation. They are meant to be used together, revisited as needed, and applied with honesty rather than urgency.

You do not need to have everything figured out to move forward.

But you do need to know what you are committing to—
and why.

Next up: SCRUBScript™

Chapter 27
SCRUBScript™

A resume is not a biography.

It is a decision document.

In healthcare, resumes are not read for aspiration or personality. They are scanned for scope, judgment, readiness, and risk. Employers are not asking whether you are motivated. They are asking whether you understand the responsibility you are stepping into—and whether you can carry it without supervision becoming a liability.

SCRUBScript™ exists to help you translate your experience **accurately**, **honestly**, and **at the right level** for where you are in your career.

Most resume advice fails clinicians because it treats resumes as static artifacts. In reality, a healthcare resume must evolve as responsibility evolves. What should be emphasized as a student is not what matters after two years, five years, or a decade in practice. When resumes fail, it is often because they are written at the wrong altitude.

SCRUBScript™ is built around progression, not polish.

Resume or CV? What Healthcare Employers Actually Expect

This is one of the most common—and most anxiety-producing—questions in healthcare.

In clinical hiring, a **resume** and a **CV** are not the same thing.

A **resume** is:

- Typically 1–2 pages (sometimes 3 for senior clinicians)
- Focused on role readiness and clinical scope
- Designed for hospitals, clinics, and health systems
- The default document for almost all clinical roles

A **CV** (curriculum vitae) is:

- Multi-page and comprehensive
- Focused on research, publications, teaching, grants, and academic service
- Used primarily for faculty roles, fellowships, and research positions

Here is the simplest rule:

If a job posting does not explicitly ask for a CV, submit a resume.

Submitting a CV when a resume is expected does not make you look more qualified. It often signals that you do not understand the hiring context. SCRUBScript™ assumes you are preparing a **resume**, unless you are pursuing an explicitly academic role.

How to Construct a Healthcare Resume

A strong healthcare resume is not creative.

It is clear.

The structure matters because hiring managers scan before they read. Confusion creates friction. Friction creates doubt.

At a minimum, your resume should include the following sections, in this order unless otherwise noted:

1 Header

2 Credentials

3 Professional Experience

4 Education

5 Licensure & Certifications

6 Additional Experience (as appropriate)

Header and Credentials

Your name should be clear and professional. Credentials matter in healthcare and should be placed prominently—either immediately after your name or directly beneath it.

This is not the place for modesty. Credentials are one of the first filters applied during resume review.

Professional Experience: How to Write Bullets That Matter

The most common mistake in healthcare resumes is vagueness.

Phrases like *"provided patient care"* or *"worked in a fast-paced environment"* communicate nothing. They force the reader to guess, and guessing creates risk.

Strong bullets answer three questions:

- **How many patients?**
- **How complex?**
- **What level of responsibility?**

For example, compare:

Provided patient care in a hospital setting.

versus

Managed care for 6–8 acute post-operative patients per shift, including assessment, medication management, care coordination, and escalation of clinical concerns to attending providers.

The second tells a hiring manager exactly what you carry.

You do not need to exaggerate. You do need to be specific.

Education, Licensure, and Certifications

Early in your career, education belongs higher on the page. As experience grows, it moves lower.

Licensure and certifications should be:

- Current
- Clearly labeled
- Easy to find

Do not make employers hunt for proof that you are qualified to practice.

Resume Evolution by Career Stage

Resumes should change as responsibility changes. A resume written at the wrong stage attracts the wrong roles.

Stage One: Student / In School

At this stage, your resume is about **proximity**, not mastery.

Employers look for:

- Clinical exposure
- Familiarity with healthcare environments
- Reliability and professionalism

Volunteering, part-time hospital work, externships, and clinical placements matter because they demonstrate intention—not independence.

Accuracy builds trust. Overreach does not.

Stage Two: New Graduate

As a new graduate, your resume should reflect **transition**, not arrival.

Employers want to see:

- Supervised responsibility
- Early clinical reasoning
- Awareness of limits
- Willingness to learn

Inflated language at this stage often creates hesitation rather than confidence.

Stage Three: Around Two Years

At roughly two years, evaluation shifts from potential to **reliability**.

This is where resumes must:

- Quantify patient load
- Describe decision-making
- Clarify independence versus escalation

Vagueness stops working here.

Stage Four: Around Five Years

By five years, employers assume competence. They assess **depth**.

Your resume should begin to show:

- Complexity tolerance
- Informal leadership
- Specialized populations
- Contributions beyond task completion

This is also where misalignment often begins to surface. Your resume should reflect the direction you are actually moving—not the one you feel pressured to pursue.

Stage Five: Ten Years and Beyond

At this stage, resumes shift from execution to **influence**.

Employers look for:

- Systems thinking
- Stability over time
- Mentorship and leadership
- The ability to steady teams and workflows

Your resume should protect future options, not lock you into an identity you've outgrown.

Why SCRUBScript™ Comes First

If your resume is written at the wrong altitude, everything downstream breaks.

You will:

- Attract roles that don't fit
- Repel opportunities that might have
- Struggle in interviews that assume a different level of readiness
- Enter negotiations from a misaligned position

SCRUBScript™ is not about polish.

It is about alignment.

When your resume accurately reflects where you are, the rest of the system works.

When it doesn't, nothing else can compensate.

Chapter 28

Writing a Current Resume

GETTING HIRED: RESUMES, INTERVIEWS, RECRUITERS & NEGOTIATIONS IN 2025

A cinematic masterclass in landing the right job — not just the first job.

Cinematic Opening: The Night Before Everything Changes

It's 9:47 PM, and your kitchen is quiet in the way kitchens only get quiet at night — refrigerator humming, dishwasher ticking its slow monotonous rhythm, a mug of lukewarm tea beside your laptop.

Your cat has planted herself on the corner of your résumé, half judging, half begging for attention. Your partner has already called twice to ask, "Are you coming to bed soon?" and been ignored twice. Spotify keeps playing lofi beats you haven't been listening to.

Tomorrow is your job interview.

Tomorrow — the day your life might tilt in a new direction.

You reread your résumé for the tenth time. You practice answers in your head. You Google the clinic one more time even though you can recite its mission statement by memory. You imagine the walk to the exam rooms, the hum of the EKG, the sterile smell of exam tables, the possibility of your badge with new credentials.

You catch your own reflection in the microwave door — tired, hopeful, terrified — and whisper:

"Okay. Let's do this."

This chapter is the blueprint for everything that comes next.

SECTION 1 — WRITING A RÉSUMÉ IN 2026: THE NEW RULES

Not cute. Not clever. Clean. Competent. Algorithm-friendly.

In 2025, your résumé is no longer read by a person first.

It's read by an algorithm — a digital bouncer standing between you and the hiring manager.

Your goal isn't to impress.

It's to **translate your clinical value into language machines and humans both understand.**

Here's how.

1. Start With a Modern Header

Make it crisp and clean:

Name (large font)

Credentials (NP Student, FNP-C, PMHNP-BC)

City + State (NOT your full address — that's outdated)

Professional email

Phone

LinkedIn (mandatory)

Optional: Personal portfolio or digital CV

2025 is digital-first.

Your résumé must be, too.

2. Your Professional Summary: The Four-Sentence Brand Statement

Forget "Objectives." They died in 2021.

Your summary should answer this:

"Who are you, clinically?"

Example:

Family Nurse Practitioner focused on evidence-based primary care with strengths in diagnostics, patient education, and chronic disease management. Former ICU nurse with proven pattern-recognition and crisis-stabilization skills. Skilled in telehealth, remote monitoring platforms, EPIC, and Cerner. Passionate about culturally competent care and improving access in underserved communities.

This tells a hiring manager more in four sentences than a full page of fluff.

3. Skills Section (Hard Skills FIRST)

Recruiters scan this in **3–6 seconds**.

Include:

- Procedures
- Diagnostics
- Populations treated
- Chronic disease management
- Acute care skills
- EHR proficiency
- Telehealth workflows
- Pharmacology strengths
- Care coordination

This is your professional fingerprint.

4. Experience Section: Show RESULTS

Old résumés list tasks.

2025 résumés show *impact.*

Bad:

- Managed chronic conditions
- Performed physical exams

Better:

- Improved A1C control in 70% of diabetic panel via medication management & education

• Performed 15–20 comprehensive exams/day with focused diagnostic reasoning

• Reduced unnecessary ED transfers through early recognition of decompensation

This is how your value becomes visible.

5. Clinical Rotations (NP Students)

Include hours + high-impact bullets.

Example:

Family Medicine | 180 Hours

• Managed acute and chronic conditions in diverse patients

• Completed well-child exams, women's health visits

• Performed suturing, splinting, joint injections (if applicable)

6. Keywords Section (2025 ATS Hack)

Use terms like:

• Evidence-based practice

• Care coordination

• Chronic disease management

• Interdisciplinary collaboration

• Patient-centered care

• Quality metrics

This helps your résumé survive the robots.

7. Format Rules for 2025

- 1 page (students), 2 pages max
- Sans-serif font
- Clean lines, no photos
- Bullet points that start with action verbs
- Save as PDF when emailing
- Save as DOCX when uploading to a hospital portal
- NO template fluff (ATS hates it)

SECTION 2 — INTERVIEWING IN 2025: HOW TO THINK OUT LOUD

You aren't being evaluated on what you know — but how you reason.

The interview room is rarely glamorous.

A desk.

Three chairs.

A half-dead fern in the corner.

A stack of résumés you pretend not to notice.

They don't want you to be perfect.

They want you to be **present, calm, clinical, and curious.**

Let's break down the canon.

1. Lead With Clinical Reasoning

Every answer should show:

1 What you noticed

2 What you thought

3 What you did

4 Why you did it

5 What happened

6 What you learned

This formula works on ANY clinical question.

2. Bring 3–5 Case Stories

Examples of:

- A diagnostic puzzle you solved
- A difficult conversation you handled
- A de-escalation you performed
- A high-risk patient you stabilized
- A safe catch
- A time you collaborated effectively

Stories prove competence more than credentials.

3. Ask Smart Questions

Clinics hire curious clinicians.

Ask:

- What's your onboarding plan for new NPs?

- How many patients per day?
- How complex is the average visit?
- Who triages?
- How are labs handled?
- How often is call?
- How does your team support burnout prevention?

These are maturity markers.

4. Manage Your Energy

They're watching:

- Are you grounded or frantic?
- Can you regulate yourself under pressure?
- Do you smile easily?
- Do you interrupt?
- Do you listen?

People hire people they want to sit next to for 8 hours.

SECTION 3 — WORKING WITH A RECRUITER

Angels or chaos gremlins — here's how to tell.

Recruiters can:

✓ Fast-track your résumé

✓ Get you interviews you'd never find alone

✓ Negotiate pay

✓ Save time

✓ Reveal hidden jobs

But they can also:

✗ Ghost you

✗ Submit your résumé without permission

✗ Pressure you into bad jobs

✗ Hide salary ranges

Let's canonize your strategy.

1. Ask if they have an exclusive relationship with the employer

If they say no, they're guessing.

If they say yes, you're in luck.

2. Ask how many NPs they've placed there

Experience matters.

3. Tell them EXACTLY what you want

- Schedule
- Salary range
- Setting
- Patient load
- Commute
- Training expectations

If you don't fire an arrow, they can't hit anything.

4. Never let a recruiter negotiate *against* you

Some will say:

"This is the best you'll get."

It rarely is.

SECTION 4 — NEGOTIATING JOB OFFERS IN 2025

This is where most NPs lose thousands — don't be one of them.

Cinematic scene:

You open the offer email.

Your stomach flips.

Is this enough?

Is this fair?

Is this insulting?

Is this your dream?

Is this a trap?

Relax.

You're about to learn how to negotiate like a seasoned clinician, not a student terrified of looking demanding.

The 2026 NP Negotiation Canon

Rule 1: Ask for the FULL offer packet

This includes:

- Base salary

- RVU (gl) structure
- Call expectations
- PTO
- CME + funding
- Sign-on bonus
- Relocation
- Malpractice: claims-made vs occurrence
- **TAIL COVERAGE** (non-negotiable to check)
- Non-compete radius
- Floating requirements
- Schedule
- Expected patient load

You cannot negotiate what you cannot see.

Rule 2: Know Your Worth (Market Bands)

You need:

- 10th percentile
- 50th percentile
- 75th percentile
- State-specific data
- Specialty-specific data

I can generate these for *any* NP specialty.

Rule 3: Never accept the first offer

Counter with:

- +10–15% base salary
- Extended CME allowance
- Loan repayment
- Reduced non-compete number
- Paid tail
- Higher sign-on bonus
- Lower patient load for the first 3 months

You won't get all of it.

But you *will* get more.

Rule 4: Use the Silence Strategy

After stating your counter:

Stop talking.

Let silence work in your favor.

Rule 5: Close with intention

Say:

"I'm enthusiastic about this role. If we can come closer on X and clarify Y, I'm ready to sign."

You're not begging.

You're collaborating.

SECTION 5 — RED FLAGS & GREEN FLAGS

Red Flags

- They won't share pay structure
- No onboarding plan
- "You'll be seeing 25–30 patients a day in month one"
- Everyone seems exhausted
- High turnover
- "We're like a family" (translation: no boundaries)
- Non-compete over 20 miles
- You can't meet the team

Green Flags

- Transparent RVU structure
- Onboarding plan of at least 8–12 weeks
- Team members who seem genuinely happy
- Access to collaborating physicians who teach, not micromanage
- Clear documentation expectations
- Reasonable patient load ramp-up
- Protected time for admin work

SECTION 6 — HOW TO KNOW WHEN TO SAY YES

You'll feel it.

You'll know it.

Your shoulders will drop, your breath will settle, your instinct will whisper,

"This is a place where I can grow."

That's alignment.

And alignment is everything.

Next up: CareerNav™

Chapter 29
CareerNav™

Most people think job searching is about effort. In healthcare, it is more accurate to say it is about location and signal. Strong candidates miss strong roles every day because they are searching in the wrong places, relying on a single platform, or assuming that hiring works the same way across organizations.

CareerNav™ is the job search system that reduces wasted motion. It shows you where healthcare jobs actually live, how to widen your search without spraying applications everywhere, and how to use networking without becoming the person who makes everyone uncomfortable.

This section has one purpose: to help you find roles that match your priorities, your constraints, and your level of readiness—so you are not interviewing for jobs you don't want and applying to roles you cannot sustain.

Where Healthcare Jobs Actually Live

If you only search job boards, you are often seeing the labor market at its noisiest. Job boards are useful, but they are not the source of truth. The source of truth is the employer.

Start here.

Hospital and health-system career sites are the most direct path to real openings, current postings, accurate requirements, and internal role descriptions that do not always appear elsewhere. These sites also help you see patterns: which departments are hiring repeatedly, which clinics are expanding, and which specialties are quietly building capacity.

Next, use professional associations.

Many healthcare roles are organized around associations that post opportunities, host career centers, and share workforce updates. Association listings tend to attract more serious applicants and often include roles that are not pushed hard on public boards. They also help you understand what is changing in the profession and where demand is rising.

Then use job boards strategically.

Indeed and LinkedIn are valuable because they cast a wide net and surface volume. But volume is not clarity. Use them to identify trends, keywords, and role titles in your region, then verify details on the employer's website before you commit time to a tailored application.

LinkedIn deserves its own category.

LinkedIn is not only a job board. It is an intelligence tool and a networking tool. Used well, it can shorten your search. Used poorly, it can create noise and anxiety. CareerNav™ treats

LinkedIn as a tool for targeted action, not a daily dopamine loop.

How to Search Without Drowning

A common mistake in healthcare job searches is applying broadly when clarity is low. That feels productive, but it often creates a second problem: too many interviews for roles you are not sure you want, followed by fatigue, followed by settling.

Start by narrowing your target using three anchors: setting, specialty, and schedule.

You do not need a perfect answer. You need a usable one. For example, "outpatient family practice, four tens, no call," or "hospitalist role, nights, defined patient volume expectations." The point is to define the boundaries that protect you.

Then build a short list of organizations.

Your goal is not to apply everywhere. Your goal is to apply where you can realistically thrive. A short list helps you recognize roles faster, tailor your materials with less effort, and track opportunities without chaos.

Finally, keep your search clean.

Job searching is mentally expensive. Set a cadence you can sustain. Two intentional sessions per week can outperform daily scrolling if the sessions are structured and focused.

Networking Without Being Weird

Networking is not schmoozing. In healthcare, networking is often nothing more than this: someone vouches that you are safe to hire.

Most opportunities come from weak ties, not best friends.

Weak ties are people who know of you, have worked adjacent to you, or share a professional context with you. They are often more useful than close friends because they connect you to circles you do not already inhabit.

CareerNav™ uses a simple approach to networking:

Start with people who already trust you, then expand outward carefully.

Friends and family can be helpful, not because they are in healthcare, but because they may know someone who is. This is the "friends-of-friends" layer. Ask for introductions, not jobs. An introduction is low pressure. A job ask creates resistance.

When you reach out, be specific.

Do not say, "Let me know if you hear of anything." That forces the other person to do the thinking. Instead, say what you are looking for in one sentence and ask for a small next step: a quick call, a point in the right direction, or a name to contact.

Your goal is not to build a massive network.

Your goal is to build a small, reliable map.

Is It OK to Send a Recruiter or Hiring Manager a LinkedIn Request?

Yes. It is acceptable to send a LinkedIn connection request to a recruiter or hiring manager, and in many cases it is smart. The key is how you do it.

Send the request with a short note. Keep it respectful, clear, and low-pressure.

You are not asking them to hire you in a message. You are signaling professionalism and making it easier for them to place you when your application crosses their screen.

A good request does three things:

It identifies the role, communicates interest, and asks for nothing heavy.

For example, you might say that you applied, you are interested, and you would value being considered if your background aligns. That is enough. The purpose is visibility, not persuasion.

Two cautions matter.

First, do not send multiple follow-ups if they do not respond. One message is professional. Repeated messages feel like pressure.

Second, do not bypass process. You still apply formally. LinkedIn is an assist, not a substitute.

Recruiters expect this. Many hiring managers do as well, especially in smaller departments or specialized services. What they do not expect is a long personal story or a high-emotion pitch. Keep it clean.

The CareerNav™ Discipline

CareerNav™ is built on one principle: targeted effort beats frantic volume.

If your search is not working, the answer is rarely "apply more."

The answer is usually one of these: you are searching in the wrong places, you are unclear about your target, your resume is not signaling readiness at the right altitude, or you are not using visibility tools correctly.

CareerNav™ gives you structure so you do not confuse activity with progress.

Next up: ApplySmart™

Chapter 30

ApplySmart™

Applying for healthcare roles is not a test of persistence.

It is a test of systems awareness.

Many strong candidates never reach a human reader—not because they are unqualified, but because their applications are filtered out long before judgment or fit can be assessed. ApplySmart™ exists to make sure your materials survive that first cut.

This section is about navigating application systems realistically, not optimistically. It explains how applicant tracking systems (ATS) work, what they screen for, and how to submit materials that pass through automation without distorting who you are.

How Applications Actually Move

Most healthcare organizations use an applicant tracking system to manage volume. These systems are designed to:

- Parse resumes into standardized fields

- Screen for required credentials
- Flag missing information
- Rank applications based on keyword alignment

They are not designed to recognize nuance, context, or potential.

This means your application is evaluated in two phases. First by a system. Then—if it survives—by a human. ApplySmart™ is about clearing the first gate so the second one can matter.

ATS-Friendly Does Not Mean Generic

A common misconception is that ATS-friendly resumes must be bland or formulaic. That is not true. What matters is structure, clarity, and alignment—not personality removal.

ATS systems struggle with:

- Complex formatting
- Tables and columns
- Graphics, icons, and text boxes
- Headers and footers with critical information
- Nonstandard fonts or symbols

If a system cannot read your resume cleanly, it cannot evaluate it fairly.

Use a simple, single-column layout. Left-align text. Use standard section headings. Save your file as a PDF only if the employer allows it; otherwise, submit a Word document.

Clarity beats cleverness every time.

Keywords Without Keyword Stuffing

ATS systems scan for keywords pulled directly from the job description. These often include:

- Role titles
- Required credentials
- Core skills
- Specialty areas
- Common clinical terms

The goal is not to repeat the job description word for word. The goal is to ensure that the language you already use to describe your work overlaps with the language the employer is screening for.

If your resume describes “primary care management” but the posting emphasizes “outpatient family medicine,” that mismatch can lower your ranking even if the work is the same.

ApplySmart™ means translating your experience into language the system recognizes—without inflating or misrepresenting it.

Completing the Application Itself

Do not assume your resume will speak for you.

Many applications require you to manually enter:

- Employment history
- Dates
- Licensure

- Certifications
- Education details

This is tedious, but it matters. Inconsistencies between your resume and application fields can flag your submission for review—or removal.

Take your time. Copy carefully. If an answer is optional but relevant, include it. Silence is often interpreted as absence.

Cover Letters: When They Matter

Cover letters are not universally required, but when they are requested, they should be brief and specific.

A strong cover letter:

- Names the role
- Signals fit with the setting or population
- Reinforces readiness rather than passion alone

Avoid generic enthusiasm. Hiring teams want reassurance, not persuasion.

If a cover letter is optional and you are applying to a highly competitive role, consider including one. If it is optional and the role is high-volume, prioritize application accuracy over additional documents.

Submitting With Intention

Applying broadly feels productive, but it often creates noise.

ApplySmart™ encourages targeted submissions. Fewer applications, better aligned, submitted cleanly and correctly, outperform high-volume approaches over time.

Before you submit, ask yourself:

- Does my resume reflect the level of responsibility this role expects?
- Does my application align with the language used in the posting?
- Am I applying because this role fits—or because I'm anxious to move?

Those questions save time and protect energy.

After You Click Submit

Once an application is submitted, resist the urge to refresh your inbox daily. Hiring timelines vary widely, especially in healthcare.

This is where visibility tools—used thoughtfully—can help. A professional LinkedIn connection request to a recruiter or hiring manager, sent after applying, can increase the likelihood that your application is seen. It does not replace the process. It supports it.

ApplySmart™ is not about beating the system. It is about understanding it well enough to move through it intact.

Next up: Intelligent Interviews™

Chapter 31
Interview Prep

Interview Prep for Nurse Practitioners

A Practical, Insider's Guide to Presenting Your Best Professional Self

You've earned the education, the clinical hours, the certification, and the confidence to step into advanced practice. But here is one truth every NP needs to hear: even the most clinically gifted practitioner can stumble if they don't know how to communicate their thinking in an interview.

This chapter distills two and a half decades of healthcare recruitment insight — the conversations that happen behind closed doors between medical directors, HR executives, and chief nursing officers — so you can walk into every NP interview with clarity, calm, and clinical precision.

Part I: Understanding What NP Interviews Actually Measure

Most candidates assume they're being evaluated on knowledge alone.

Not true.

NP interviews assess:

- **Clinical reasoning**
- **Communication style**
- **Professional maturity**
- **Team compatibility**
- **Safety awareness**
- **Self-awareness**
- **Alignment with the practice environment**

Hiring managers want to know:

1. *Can you think?*

2. *Are you safe?*

3. *Will you thrive here?*

4. *Can you practice independently without being isolated?*

Part II: The Five Categories of NP Interview Questions

1. Clinical Judgment

Expect case-based questions. They're not looking for perfection — they're looking for your process.

Common prompts:

- "Tell me how you approach a patient with abdominal pain."

- "What is your differential for shortness of breath?"
- "How do you decide when to order imaging?"

Answer using:

- Red flags
- Pathway or algorithm
- Labs or imaging
- First-line treatments
- Safety plan & follow-up

They want to see if your reasoning is structured, safe, and teachable.

2. Communication & Patient Interaction

Advanced practice means advanced communication.

You may be asked:

- "Describe a time you had to explain a complex diagnosis in plain language."
- "How would you handle a patient who wants an antibiotic that isn't indicated?"
- "How do you build trust quickly with new patients?"

Show that you balance clarity, compassion, and boundaries.

3. Collaboration & Practice Culture Fit

NPs are part of intricate clinical ecosystems.

Sample questions:

• “Tell me about a time you collaborated with a physician.”

• “How do you respond when a colleague disagrees with your plan?”

• “Describe an ideal supervisory relationship.”

The goal: Show that you are independent, but not isolated.

Confident, not rigid.

Collaborative, not deferential.

4. Stress, Safety, and Ethical Situations

These questions reveal your grounding under pressure.

Examples:

• “How do you prioritize when you have three patients waiting and one is deteriorating?”

• “Tell me about a time you were unsure of a diagnosis — what did you do?”

• “Describe an ethical dilemma you navigated.”

They want to hear:

• Safety first

• Clear communication

• A willingness to escalate early

• Humility without insecurity

• Sound boundaries

5. Fit, Values, and Alignment

This is where you become unforgettable.

Expect:

- "Why do you want to work here?"
- "What gives you the most satisfaction in practice?"
- "What kind of environment supports your best work?"
- "Where do you see your practice evolving?"

This is your SCRUBfit™ moment — demonstrating how your wiring, pace, and professional philosophy align with their practice.

Sample answer:

I provide my best care in environments that balance autonomy with support, where communication is open and clinicians can work at the top of their license. I'm intentional about alignment because the right environment allows me to bring my full clinical judgment and presence to every patient.

Part III: How to Prepare Before the Interview

1. Know the Organization

At minimum, research:

- The patient population
- Practice mission and values
- Clinical model (team-based? value-based?)
- Recent growth or service expansions
- Quality rankings or recognitions

This allows you to speak intelligently — and avoids the dreaded "generic answers."

2. Understand the Expectations

You should be ready to discuss:

- Average patient volume
- Administrative time
- Call or weekend rotations
- Panel management expectations
- EMR used
- Performance metrics

Surprises after hiring are the number one cause of early NP turnover.

3. Prepare Your Clinical Stories

Have 5–7 polished examples ready — real, specific, and demonstrating both skill and judgment.

Include:

- A complex case you managed
- A time you collaborated effectively
- A moment you caught something early
- A time you escalated care appropriately
- A situation that changed you
- A time you advocated for a patient

• A moment you balanced autonomy and uncertainty

Use the **Situation → Assessment → Action → Outcome** structure.

4. Prepare High-Quality Questions for Them

Strong candidates ask strong questions.

Examples:

• "What does success look like in the first 90 days?"

• "How do new NPs receive support during onboarding?"

• "How is clinical decision-making shared among the team?"

• "What are the biggest challenges facing this patient population?"

• "How does the practice measure and evaluate quality?"

Never end an interview with: *No questions. I think we covered everything.*

That sinks candidates instantly.

Part IV: Interview Day — How to Present Your Best Clinical Self

1. Arrive Early Enough to Observe the Culture

Notice:

• How the front desk greets patients

• How team members speak to one another

• How rushed or calm the pace seems

Your practice environment matters as much as your paycheck.

2. Communicate Clearly and Slowly

Your interviewer is assessing:

- Your clarity
- Your organization
- Your confidence
- Your teachability

Speak like you would to a patient:

Grounded, calm, measured.

3. If You Don't Know Something, Say So

The right answer is:

"Based on what I know, here is how I would approach it. Before finalizing a plan, I would consult X or review Y."

Safety always outranks ego.

Part V: After the Interview

1. Send a Thoughtful Follow-Up

Keep it short but personal to the conversation.

2. Reflect Honestly

Ask yourself:

- Could I see myself thriving here?
- Do I trust the culture?
- Does the pace match my wiring?
- Did the environment feel supportive?

• Does this practice align with who I am becoming?

This is not just a job — it's a long-term professional identity decision.

Final Words for Every Future NP

Your interview is not a test of perfection.

It is a window into how you think, how you care, and how you practice.

Walk in with:

• Clinical clarity

• Measured communication

• Solid reasoning

• Genuine curiosity

• Professional confidence

• Alignment awareness

You are not selling yourself.

You are showing the interviewer who you already are as a clinician.

And Mason — this chapter now fits beautifully alongside your certification/licensure, credentialing, financial landscape, and career guidance chapters for ScrubTales™: Nurse Practitioner.

Next up: Intelligent Interviews™

Chapter 32

Intelligent Interviews™

Healthcare interviews are not conversations.

They are assessments.

They are designed to evaluate judgment, decision-making, accountability, and risk—not charm, enthusiasm, or how badly you want the job. Intelligent Interviews™ exists to help you understand what interviewers are actually testing so you can respond with clarity rather than performance.

Many clinicians leave interviews feeling uncertain—not because they answered poorly, but because they misunderstood the purpose of the questions. Behavioral interviews are not about storytelling. They are about evidence.

What Interviewers Are Really Assessing

In healthcare, interviews focus on three underlying questions:

- Can this person make sound decisions under pressure?
- Do they understand the limits of their role?

- Will they function safely and predictably inside our system?

Questions are rarely framed this directly. Instead, they are embedded in prompts about past experiences, difficult situations, conflict, or mistakes. These questions are designed to surface how you think when protocols end and judgment begins.

Intelligent Interviews™ shifts your focus from "How do I impress?" to "How do I demonstrate readiness?"

Behavioral Interviewing, Decoded

Behavioral interviewing is built on a simple premise: past behavior is the best available predictor of future behavior.

When an interviewer asks you to describe a challenging case, a conflict with a colleague, or a time something went wrong, they are not grading your outcome. They are listening for:

- Situational awareness
- Clinical reasoning
- Accountability
- Learning and adaptation

Strong answers describe what happened, what you noticed, what you decided, and what you would do differently next time. Weak answers stay vague, shift blame, or rush to resolution without reflection.

You do not need dramatic stories. You need honest ones.

Answering With Judgment, Not Just Experience

A common mistake is overemphasizing action while underexplaining reasoning.

For example, saying “I escalated the issue to the attending” is less informative than explaining why escalation was appropriate at that moment. Interviewers want to hear how you weigh risk, recognize limits, and choose next steps.

When answering, anchor your response in three elements:

- What information you had
- What you were responsible for
- How you decided what to do

This structure demonstrates judgment without sounding defensive or rehearsed.

Talking About Mistakes and Uncertainty

Nearly every healthcare interview includes a question about mistakes, conflict, or difficult outcomes. These questions are uncomfortable by design.

The goal is not to see whether you are flawless. It is to see whether you are honest, reflective, and safe.

Avoid minimizing errors or framing yourself as a victim of circumstances. At the same time, do not catastrophize. Describe what happened, what you learned, and how your practice changed as a result.

Mature answers show accountability without self-punishment.

Questions You Should Be Prepared For

While no two interviews are identical, many healthcare interviews return to similar themes:

- Managing competing priorities
- Handling uncertainty
- Navigating conflict
- Recognizing limits
- Responding to feedback
- Working within constraints

Preparation does not mean memorizing scripts. It means identifying experiences that illustrate your judgment and being ready to discuss them calmly and clearly.

Questions You Should Ask

Interviews are also an opportunity to assess fit. The questions you ask signal what you value and how you think.

Strong questions explore:

- Expectations for decision-making autonomy
- Support and supervision structures
- Patient volume and acuity
- Team dynamics
- Measures of success in the role

Avoid questions that focus only on perks or schedule early in the process. Those matter, but timing matters too.

Pre-Interview Intelligence

Before any interview, conduct basic organizational research. This is not optional.

Review the organization's website. Look up recent news. Search for public information about lawsuits, union activity, leadership changes, or restructuring. Understand the setting you are stepping into.

This preparation helps you ask better questions and recognize misalignment early.

The Goal of Intelligent Interviews™

The goal is not to win the interview.

The goal is to decide whether this role deserves you.

When you understand how interviews work, you can stop performing and start evaluating. That shift protects you from accepting roles that look good on paper but fail in practice.

Intelligent Interviews™ helps you enter interviews prepared, grounded, and clear—so that whatever decision follows is one you can stand behind.

Next up: Terms of Care™

Chapter 33

Must Have - Saying Thank You

The Power of the Post-Interview Thank-You (Especially for Nurse Practitioners)

Sending a thank-you note after an interview isn't a courtesy — it's a clinical skill. It shows emotional intelligence, respect, and professionalism, the same qualities employers expect from a high-functioning NP. In today's competitive market, where every candidate may have the same certifications, what sets you apart is how you communicate and connect. A thoughtful thank-you keeps you top-of-mind, reinforces why you're the right fit, and signals that you follow through — an essential trait in advanced practice.

Personal Advice

Even if you walk out of an interview feeling certain the position isn't the right fit, be professional and send a thank-you note anyway. Healthcare is moving at the speed of mergers and acquisitions, and today's "not-for-me" organization may become your employer tomorrow. The leader you just met could easily become your next medical director, collaborating partner, or boss through a merger, acquisition, or network shift. Protect your reputation, keep doors open, and never burn bridges — this is a small, small world.

Whether you email immediately, send a handwritten note later, or both, your message becomes part of the impression you leave behind. And in healthcare, impressions matter.

Don't forget the Recruiter

Never forget to thank the recruiter who reached out to you, advocated for you, and coordinated your interview. Recruiters are often the quiet power players in the hiring process, and you never know when the perfect opportunity may come through them in the future. Make yourself memorable in a positive way: return their calls and emails promptly, be courteous, be responsive, and treat every interaction as part of the interview.

Do not be naïve and assume the recruiter has limited influence. In reality, they often have extremely strong relationships with hiring managers and clinical leaders — sometimes stronger than candidates realize. And remember this: the recruiter is often the one conducting your reference checks. Reference checking is a skill, and experienced recruiters know how to ask the right questions, interpret tone, and read between the lines. Their impressions of you — and the impressions they gather about you — matter.

When recruiting, my top priority was always patient safety and patient experience. If I wouldn't feel comfortable seeing you as a patient myself, your résumé typically never reached the hiring manager's desk. Recruiters have a vote — and often an important one. Treat them with the respect, gratitude, and professionalism that reflects well on you now *and* protects opportunities later.

Email Thank-You Note (NP Version)

Subject: Thank You for the Opportunity

Hi [Interviewer's Name],

Thank you so much for taking the time to speak with me today. I truly enjoyed learning more about the role, your clinical team, and the culture you've built. The way you described your approach to patient care strongly resonated with me, and our conversation reinforced how well my background in [your NP specialty, e.g., FNP, ACNP, PMHNP] aligns with your needs.

I appreciate your transparency, your insight into the department's goals, and the warmth you brought to the conversation. Please let me know if I can provide anything additional as you move forward in your decision-making process. I'm very excited about the possibility of contributing to the team and supporting excellent patient outcomes.

Warmly,

[Your Name], [Credentials]

Handwritten Thank-You Note (Short & Impactful)

Dear [Interviewer's Name],

Thank you again for the opportunity to interview for the Nurse Practitioner position. I appreciated our conversation and especially enjoyed hearing about your team's vision for patient care. I would be honored to contribute my skills, compassion, and commitment to clinical excellence to your organization.

Warmest regards,

[Your Name]

Tip:

Send the email within 24 hours.

Send the handwritten note within 48–72 hours — it becomes your memorable "extra touch."

Quick Text-Friendly Thank-You

If appropriate (only when you've been texting with the hiring manager or recruiter):

Hi [Name], thank you again for today — I really enjoyed our conversation and learning more about the NP role. I'm excited about the opportunity and appreciate your time!

Chapter 34

Terms of Care™

Accepting a healthcare job is not a single decision.

It is an agreement.

Terms of Care™ exists to help you understand what you are actually agreeing to when you say yes—not just in compensation, but in expectations, workload, boundaries, and sustainability.

Many clinicians approach negotiation cautiously, or avoid it altogether, out of fear of appearing difficult or ungrateful. Others focus narrowly on salary without understanding the broader structure of the offer. Both approaches miss the point.

Negotiation in healthcare is not about leverage.

It is about clarity.

What a Job Offer Really Contains

A job offer is a bundle of terms, not a number. Salary is only one component, and often not the most important one.

Most offers include:

- Base compensation
- Benefits
- Schedule and call expectations
- Productivity targets
- Scope and autonomy
- Support structures
- Non-compete or restrictive clauses
- Onboarding expectations

These elements interact. A higher salary paired with unsustainable workload is not a better offer. A modest salary paired with strong support and realistic expectations may be.

Terms of Care™ teaches you to evaluate offers as systems, not line items.

Understanding Total Rewards

Healthcare organizations often refer to compensation packages as **Total Rewards.** This term can feel abstract, but it reflects a real financial reality: benefits typically cost employers approximately **30 percent** of base salary.

Total Rewards may include:

- Health, dental, and vision insurance
- Retirement contributions
- Paid time off

- Continuing education funds
- Licensing and certification support
- Loan repayment assistance
- Malpractice coverage
- Disability and life insurance

Understanding this context matters. It helps you interpret offers accurately and frame negotiations realistically. When you understand what the organization is investing, conversations become clearer and less adversarial.

What Is Negotiable—and What Usually Isn't

Not every element of an offer is negotiable, but more is flexible than many clinicians assume.

Often negotiable:

- Start date
- Schedule structure
- PTO accrual or timing
- Continuing education support
- Loan repayment contributions
- Onboarding timeline

Less often negotiable:

- Core benefits packages
- Standard malpractice coverage

• Organizational policies tied to union agreements or systemwide rules

Asking thoughtful questions is not the same as demanding changes. Negotiation is information gathering first, adjustment second.

The Long Payback

Loan repayment deserves special attention because it shapes long-term flexibility.

Student debt does not simply affect monthly budgets. It influences:

• Job mobility

• Willingness to tolerate misalignment

• Ability to pivot or reduce hours later

Some employers offer loan repayment assistance, either directly or through state and federal programs. Others structure sign-on bonuses that can be applied to debt, though these often come with repayment obligations if you leave early.

Understanding the difference between immediate cash and long-term relief matters. Terms of Care™ encourages you to look beyond the first year and ask how this role supports—or constrains—your future options.

Boundaries Are Part of the Agreement

One of the most overlooked aspects of negotiation is boundary clarity.

This includes:

- Patient volume expectations
- Call coverage
- After-hours responsibilities
- Documentation expectations
- Coverage during absences

If these are unclear at the offer stage, they rarely become clearer later. Terms of Care™ treats boundary-setting as an act of professionalism, not conflict.

Saying Yes, Saying No, and Asking for Time

You do not need to accept an offer immediately.

It is reasonable to:

- Ask for time to review
- Request clarification in writing
- Discuss concerns respectfully
- Decline an offer that does not align

Choosing not to accept a role is not a failure. It is a decision in service of sustainability.

The Purpose of Terms of Care™

This section is not about “winning” a negotiation.

It is about entering an agreement with open eyes.

When terms are clear, responsibility is shared. When they are vague, the burden often falls on the clinician.

Terms of Care™ exists to help you protect your future self—before momentum and obligation make that harder.

Next up: The 90-Day Pathway™

Chapter 35

The 90-Day Pathway™

The first ninety days in a healthcare role are not a warm-up.

They are a signal-detection period.

This is when expectations crystallize, support structures reveal themselves, and early misalignment becomes visible—often long before anyone names it out loud. The 90-Day Pathway™ exists to help you stabilize yourself in the role *before* doubt hardens into regret or exhaustion.

Many clinicians assume that discomfort in the early months is simply part of learning. Some of it is. But some of it is information. The challenge is knowing the difference.

What the First 90 Days Are Really For

Organizations often frame onboarding as orientation, training, or assimilation. From your perspective, the first ninety days serve a different purpose.

They answer three critical questions:

• Is the reality of this role consistent with how it was described?

• Do I have the support I was told I would have?

• Can I see myself sustaining this work once the learning curve flattens?

The goal is not to prove yourself.

The goal is to assess fit while adjustments are still possible.

Stabilization Before Optimization

One of the most common mistakes clinicians make early is trying to optimize too soon. They take on extra patients, volunteer for additional responsibilities, or push themselves to "keep up" before they understand the system they are in.

The 90-Day Pathway™ prioritizes stabilization:

• Learning workflows before changing them

• Understanding escalation pathways before stretching autonomy

• Observing team dynamics before inserting solutions

Early overperformance can create long-term expectations that are difficult to reset.

Week 1–30: Learning the Real Job

The first month is about observation and pattern recognition.

Pay attention to:

• How decisions are actually made

- Who is available when questions arise
- What happens when things go wrong
- How documentation expectations match reality

Notice where support is consistent and where it is conditional. These details matter more than formal policies.

Days 31–60: Pressure Reveals Structure

As novelty fades, pressure increases.

This is when patient volume rises, supervision often loosens, and unspoken expectations surface. Pay attention to how you feel at the end of the day—not just physically, but cognitively.

Ask yourself:

- Am I thinking about work after I leave?
- Do I feel clear or scattered?
- Are questions welcomed or tolerated?

These signals help you distinguish normal adjustment from structural misalignment.

Days 61–90: Early Course Correction

By the third month, you have enough information to act.

This does not mean making dramatic decisions. It means making *small, timely adjustments*:

- Clarifying expectations
- Asking for feedback

- Resetting boundaries
- Requesting additional support where needed

Waiting too long allows patterns to solidify. Early conversations are easier than later confrontations.

What to Document for Yourself

During the first ninety days, keep informal notes—not for performance reviews, but for clarity.

Track:

- Moments of confidence
- Moments of strain
- Questions that repeat
- Situations that drain you disproportionately

These notes become invaluable if you later reassess fit, renegotiate terms, or consider next moves.

The Role of Doubt

Doubt is not a failure signal. It is information.

The question is whether doubt decreases as competence increases, or whether it persists because the structure itself is misaligned. The 90-Day Pathway™ helps you observe that pattern without rushing to judgment.

Why This Section Matters

Many clinicians exit roles within the first year not because they were incapable, but because early misalignment was ignored until it became untenable.

The first ninety days are your window for clarity.

Use them intentionally.

Next up: Shortage Indicator™

Chapter 36

Shortage Indicator™

Demand matters—but it is not the same thing as fit.

The Shortage Indicator™ exists to help you understand *why* Nurse Practitioners are in demand, *where* that demand is concentrated, and *what tradeoffs* often accompany shortage-driven hiring. High demand can create opportunity, but it can also obscure risk if it is misunderstood.

This section is not about convincing you that you will find a job. In most markets, Nurse Practitioners will. The more important question is **what kind of job demand is being created—and at what cost to the people filling it**.

What a Shortage Actually Signals

A shortage does not automatically mean a role is desirable. It means one or more of the following is true:

- Demand for services is increasing
- Fewer clinicians are entering the role

• Clinicians are leaving faster than they are replaced

• Working conditions make retention difficult

• Compensation has not kept pace with workload or responsibility

Shortages are signals. They tell a story about system stress.

Understanding *which* of these factors is driving demand in your region helps you interpret job postings more intelligently.

Where Demand for Nurse Practitioners Is Strongest

Shortage patterns for Nurse Practitioners often cluster around:

• Primary care

• Rural and underserved areas

• High-volume outpatient settings

• Specialties with heavy call or documentation burden

These roles may offer:

• Faster hiring

• Sign-on incentives

• Loan repayment support

• Greater autonomy earlier

They may also come with:

• Higher patient volume

• Thinner support structures

- Broader scope expectations
- Less protected learning time

Neither list is inherently good or bad. The tradeoff is the point.

Shortage Incentives: Read Them Carefully

Incentives often appear where pressure is highest.

Sign-on bonuses, relocation packages, and loan repayment programs can be helpful—but they are rarely free. They are usually tied to time commitments, repayment clauses, or workload expectations that should be understood fully before acceptance.

A role offering aggressive incentives may be a strong opportunity—or it may be compensating for structural strain. The Shortage Indicator™ helps you pause long enough to tell the difference.

Shortage Does Not Equal Sustainability

One of the most common mistakes clinicians make is assuming that strong demand guarantees long-term viability. In reality, some of the most consistently open roles are open *because* they are difficult to sustain.

Ask yourself:

- Why does this role turn over?
- What happens to the people who leave?
- How long do clinicians typically stay?
- What support exists to make the role viable beyond the first year?

Demand without durability is a warning sign, not a selling point.

Using the Shortage Indicator™ Wisely

The Shortage Indicator™ should inform your decision, not drive it.

High demand can give you leverage in negotiations, flexibility in timing, and access to roles that might otherwise be difficult to enter. It should not pressure you into accepting misalignment simply because opportunities are abundant.

Shortages create options.

Fit determines outcomes.

What Comes Next

Understanding market demand is only part of the picture. Financial realities often exert equal or greater pressure on decision-making—especially when debt, compensation structures, and long-term tradeoffs are involved.

Next up: Financial Landscape™

Chapter 37
Financial Landscape™

Money is rarely the reason people enter healthcare.

It is often the reason they stay longer than they should—or leave sooner than they planned.

Financial Landscape™ exists to bring realism into a space that is often dominated by averages, projections, and optimism. This section is not about maximizing income. It is about understanding how compensation, costs, and debt interact over time so you can make decisions that remain viable as circumstances change.

For Nurse Practitioners, financial pressure tends to show up gradually. The numbers may look acceptable on paper, but the lived reality can feel tighter than expected once taxes, benefits, loan payments, and time costs are accounted for.

Understanding Pay Beyond the Headline

Salary figures are often discussed as ranges or national averages. These numbers are useful only in context.

What matters more than the headline salary is:

- Take-home pay after taxes and deductions
- Cost of living in the region
- Schedule demands tied to compensation
- Productivity expectations embedded in the role

Two roles with identical salaries can feel dramatically different depending on patient volume, call responsibilities, and documentation burden. Financial Landscape™ encourages you to look past the number and ask how the money is earned.

Productivity, RVUs, and Incentive Structures

Many Nurse Practitioner roles include productivity components, often tied to RVUs or similar metrics. These structures can reward efficiency, but they can also increase pressure if expectations are unclear.

Before accepting a role with productivity incentives, understand:

- How productivity is measured
- What support exists to meet targets
- Whether targets adjust during onboarding
- How compensation changes if targets are missed

Incentives that look generous can become stressful if the system does not support sustainable throughput.

The Long Payback

Loan repayment deserves focused attention because it shapes flexibility over time.

Student debt affects more than monthly budgets. It influences:

- Willingness to tolerate misalignment
- Ability to reduce hours later
- Freedom to pivot roles or settings
- Timing of major life decisions

Some employers offer direct loan repayment assistance or participate in state and federal programs. Others structure sign-on bonuses that can be applied to debt, often with repayment clauses if you leave early.

Understanding the difference between immediate cash and long-term relief matters. A bonus can feel helpful in the short term, but loan repayment reduces long-term drag on your options.

Financial Landscape™ encourages you to model scenarios, not just accept offers. Ask what your financial life looks like in year one, year three, and year five—not just at signing.

Hidden Costs and Time Tradeoffs

Compensation is only one side of the ledger. Time is the other.

Consider:

- Commute length
- Unpaid documentation time

- Call recovery
- Schedule inflexibility
- Emotional recovery after demanding days

These costs rarely appear in contracts, but they affect sustainability just as much as salary.

Why Financial Clarity Protects Fit

Financial pressure has a way of narrowing choices. When money feels tight, it becomes harder to leave misaligned roles, renegotiate terms, or slow down when needed.

Clarity creates options.

Financial Landscape™ is not about telling you what to accept. It is about helping you understand the consequences of acceptance before they accumulate.

Next up: Next Moves™ — Not Every Pivot Is an Exit

Chapter 38
Job Market and Salary Data

The job market for Nurse Practitioners isn't just "good." It is structurally strong, and it has been for years, because it is being pushed by forces bigger than any single hospital system: physician shortages, an aging population, expanding chronic disease, mental health demand, and a healthcare economy that is trying to do more care with fewer bottlenecks. The result is a profession that keeps growing, keeps diversifying into new settings, and keeps offering leverage to clinicians who understand how to read the market instead of guessing.

According to the U.S. Bureau of Labor Statistics, Nurse Practitioner employment is projected to grow about **40% from 2024 to 2034**, and the field is expected to produce roughly **32,700 openings per year** on average. That growth rate is not a motivational quote. It is a pressure signal. It means demand will keep expanding, but it also means employers will keep experimenting with productivity expectations, care models, and staffing mixes. In other words:

opportunity is real, and so is the risk of getting absorbed into an environment that looks great on paper but quietly drains you in practice.

What the demand actually looks like on the ground often depends on where you stand and what you practice. Primary care, geriatrics, psychiatry, urgent care, and acute care continue to pull strongly, but "high demand" does not always mean "high support." Some of the hottest markets are hot because they are growing quickly and cannot staff fast enough, and that can create chaotic onboarding, aggressive patient volumes, and unclear scope boundaries. The goal isn't just to find a job. The goal is to find a job market pocket where the demand is strong **and** the practice conditions allow you to stay safe, steady, and sustainable.

Salary reality: the number is only the start. BLS data puts the **median NP pay around $129,210 (2024)**, but that single figure hides the real story: pay varies sharply by geography, specialty, setting, call expectations, and productivity structure. A hospital-based NP role may pay differently than outpatient, a psychiatric NP role may behave differently than primary care, and a "great salary" can become mediocre fast if you are doing large amounts of uncompensated inbox work, charting at night, or taking call without real recovery time.

That is why compensation should be evaluated as a **package**, not a number. When you read an offer, your brain will naturally lock onto base salary because it feels concrete. Train yourself to widen the lens immediately. Look at total rewards: CME funding and paid days, licensing and DEA costs covered, malpractice type and tail coverage, loan repayment, retirement match, productivity/RVU structure, admin time, call pay, schedule flexibility, and—most overlooked—how portal volume and documentation expectations are handled. A lower base can outperform a higher base if the structure protects your time and your nervous system.

Where the strongest leverage often lives is in underserved and rural access markets, community health environments, and systems that are actively expanding care. These settings can come with meaningful incentives—loan repayment programs, sign-on bonuses, relocation support, schedule creativity—but they can also come with thinner resources. The correct move is not to romanticize "incentives," and it is not to fear them either. The correct move is to ask better questions: What is the patient complexity? Who is triaging? How is after-hours handled? What does success look like in the first 90 days? How protected is your admin time? In high-need markets, the wrong contract can burn you out quickly. The right one can change your life.

Use demand signals as a negotiation tool, not as a fantasy. When job growth is strong, employers compete. Sometimes they compete transparently with pay; more often they compete quietly through schedule, support, autonomy, and training. Your negotiation power increases when you show that you understand the market and that you are evaluating fit, not begging for approval. This is where you connect the dots across the book: Job market strength gives you options, and options protect alignment. You do not negotiate to "win." You negotiate to build a structure you can live inside without slowly resenting your own success.

Your bottom-line market rule is simple: if an employer cannot articulate patient volume expectations, onboarding structure, documentation norms, and support resources with clarity, they are telling you the truth without saying it. The market may be strong, but your safety still depends on choosing conditions that match how you are wired, how you practice, and what you need to thrive.

Data hygiene: stay current without spiraling. Use BLS for baseline wage and outlook context, then verify local reality by checking multiple sources: state and metro pay patterns, specialty differences, and local employer ranges. Most importantly, validate the numbers in conversation with real humans—recruiters who place NPs in that exact market, NPs working in that specialty, and clinical leaders who can explain ramp-up expectations. The goal is not to become an economist. The goal is to become a calm, informed decision-maker who refuses to confuse "high demand" with "high fit."

If you want, I'll do this next in the same "install and lock" style: I'll generate (1) a one-page "Market Questions Checklist" that plugs directly into your interview/negotiation sequence, and (2) a short "Salary Bands Without the Lies" subsection that stays BLS-grounded but still reads like lived reality.

Market Questions Checklist™ — Reading the NP Job Market Like a Professional

Before you accept an offer, negotiate compensation, or relocate for a role, you need more than salary data. You need **signal clarity**. This checklist turns "job market demand" into concrete, answerable questions that protect you from misalignment disguised as opportunity.

Use this checklist **during interviews, recruiter conversations, and final offer review**. If an employer cannot answer these clearly, that itself is data.

Demand & Stability Signals

- Why is this position open?
  - Growth
  - Turnover
  - Expansion into new services
  - Replacement for departure
- How long has this role been open?
- How many NPs have been hired here in the past 12–24 months?
- How long do NPs typically stay in this role?

High demand + high turnover is not a win. It's a warning.

Patient Volume & Complexity

- What is the expected patient volume:
  - First 30 days
  - First 90 days
  - At full productivity
- What percentage of visits are:
  - Acute
  - Chronic

◦ Complex / multi-comorbidity

- Who triages patient complexity?
- What happens when complexity exceeds visit time?

Volume without triage equals burnout.

Onboarding & Ramp-Up

- Is there a formal onboarding plan?
- How long is protected onboarding?
- Are patient numbers capped during ramp-up?
- Who is clinically available when questions arise?
- How often are new NPs reviewed during the first 90 days?

"No set onboarding" means you are the onboarding plan.

Documentation & Admin Load

- What EHR is used?
- Are templates standardized or clinician-built?
- How much admin time is protected weekly?
- How is inbox / portal work handled?
- Is portal time counted toward productivity?

Unpaid cognitive labor erodes compensation quietly.

Support Structure

- Who supports:

◦ Prior authorizations

- Referrals
- Results management
- Patient education follow-up

- How many MAs / RNs per provider?
- Who covers when you are out?

Support ratios matter as much as salary.

Call, Coverage & Boundaries

- Is call required?
- How often?
- Paid or unpaid?
- What happens if a patient issue escalates after hours?
- Who is legally responsible?

Call without clarity is a liability.

Growth & Longevity

- What does success look like at:
  - 6 months
  - 1 year
  - 3 years
- Are there pathways for:
  - Schedule flexibility
  - Specialty focus

  - Leadership
  - Teaching
- Why do people stay here?

Strong markets reward clinicians who last.

Alignment Check

- Does this environment reward speed or judgment?
- Are NPs trusted — or tolerated?
- Does leadership understand NP scope?
- Can you imagine practicing here **without shrinking yourself**?

If the market is strong, you don't have to settle.

Salary Bands Without the Lies™ — What NP Pay Really Means

Salary data is helpful — but dangerous — when it's taken at face value. The Nurse Practitioner market looks lucrative on paper, yet many NPs quietly under-earn once workload, documentation, call, and unpaid labor are factored in. This section teaches you how to read salary bands **as systems**, not numbers.

Baseline Reality (Context, Not Promise)

National data places median NP compensation around the high-$120Ks range, with variation driven by:

- Specialty
- Region

- Practice setting
- Productivity expectations
- Autonomy level

This is **context**, not entitlement.

The Three Salary Bands That Matter

Instead of asking "What do NPs make?", ask where **this job** sits in the market.

Lower Market Band

- Often entry-level or high-support roles
- Strong onboarding
- Lower patient volume
- Better boundaries
- Often worth it early in career

Mid-Market Band

- Most common
- Moderate productivity expectations
- Requires negotiation to protect time
- Where alignment matters most

Upper Market Band

- High demand specialties or locations
- Often productivity-driven
- Can hide:

  - Aggressive volumes
  - Weak support
  - Burnout risk

High pay without structural protection is borrowed energy.

What Actually Moves Compensation

Salary shifts when one or more of these increase:

- Patient volume
- Case complexity
- Autonomy
- Call responsibility
- RVU expectations
- Geographic scarcity

If compensation doesn't rise when responsibility rises, you are subsidizing the system.

Total Compensation (The Part Most NPs Miss)

Evaluate offers using **total reward value**, not base pay:

- Base salary
- RVU or productivity structure
- CME funding + paid CME days
- Loan repayment
- Sign-on bonus
- Relocation

- PTO
- Malpractice type + tail
- Admin time
- Schedule control

A “lower” salary with strong structure can outperform a higher salary that costs you your evenings, weekends, and nervous system.

Early-Career Pay Trap

New NPs often under-negotiate because:

- They fear being seen as demanding
- They underestimate market leverage
- They overvalue prestige
- They undervalue sustainability

Strong markets allow you to ask for:

- Lower initial patient load
- Extended onboarding
- Paid admin time
- Education funding
- Loan repayment
- Tail coverage

You do not need to earn everything at once — but you must not give everything away.

The Alignment Rule

The best-paid NP is not the one with the highest salary.

It is the one who can:

- Practice safely
- Recover fully
- Stay curious
- Stay human
- Stay long enough to grow

Job markets rise and fall.

Alignment compounds.

Chapter 39

Long Term Career Growth and Entrepreneurship

How Nurse Practitioners Build Careers That Expand Instead of Shrink

Early in your career, success as a Nurse Practitioner often looks like competence.

Later, it looks like sustainability.

What most NP programs prepare you for is *entry*: passing boards, landing a job, surviving the learning curve. What they rarely prepare you for is what happens after year three, year seven, or year fifteen—when the role is no longer new, the responsibility is familiar, and the question quietly shifts from *"Can I do this?"* to *"How long do I want to do this like this?"*

Long-term career growth for NPs is not about climbing a ladder. It is about **expanding options**—so your work can evolve as your identity, energy, and life circumstances change. This chapter is about how Nurse Practitioners build careers that **widen over time instead of narrowing**, and how entrepreneurship—broadly defined—becomes one of the most powerful tools for alignment and longevity.

The Hidden Career Arc of Nurse Practitioners

Most NP careers follow one of three trajectories:

Some **plateau**.

The role stabilizes, but growth slows. Pay stagnates. Curiosity dulls. The work becomes predictable—but heavy.

Some **burn**.

Responsibility increases without structural protection. Patient load grows. Documentation spills into nights. Emotional reserves thin. These clinicians are capable, respected, and quietly exhausted.

Some **expand**.

Their scope deepens, their influence widens, and their work adapts to their life rather than competing with it.

The difference is not talent.

It is **intentional design**.

Career Growth Is Not Always Vertical

Healthcare often frames advancement as upward movement: titles, leadership roles, administration. But for many NPs, the most meaningful growth is **horizontal or diagonal**.

Growth may look like:

- Moving from generalist to niche specialist

- Reducing volume while increasing complexity
- Trading speed for depth
- Shifting from full-time clinical work to a blended portfolio
- Teaching, mentoring, or consulting alongside practice
- Building something that exists beyond your patient panel

None of these are exits. They are **evolutions**.

Entrepreneurship for Nurse Practitioners (Redefined)

Entrepreneurship does not only mean opening a brick-and-mortar clinic.

For NPs, entrepreneurship means **owning part of how you create value** instead of trading all of your time for someone else's system.

That ownership can take many forms:

- Independent or group practice (where allowed)
- Telehealth services
- Specialty clinics (women's health, mental health, aesthetics, wellness)
- Consulting for healthcare organizations
- Education, training, or curriculum development
- Content creation, writing, or speaking
- Clinical leadership in startup or innovation spaces
- Side practices that grow into primary work

Entrepreneurship is not about leaving care.

It is about **shaping care on your terms.**

Why Entrepreneurship Matters for Longevity

Clinical work is meaningful—but it is also finite.

Your hands, focus, and emotional bandwidth are not unlimited resources. Over time, careers that rely exclusively on high-volume direct care often become brittle. One injury, one life shift, one change in tolerance—and the entire structure strains.

Entrepreneurial pathways create:

- Income diversification
- Schedule flexibility
- Creative engagement
- Cognitive variety
- Reduced dependence on a single employer
- Psychological safety through optionality

Optionality is not greed.

It is resilience.

The Timing Myth

Many NPs believe entrepreneurship is something you do *after* you've "paid your dues."

In reality, the best time to **start thinking** entrepreneurially is early—before burnout forces the question.

You do not need to act immediately.

You need to **notice patterns**:

- What patients do you gravitate toward?
- What problems energize you?
- What parts of care feel draining versus generative?
- Where do colleagues already come to you for help?
- What frustrations make you think, *"There has to be a better way"*?

Those signals are the raw material of future growth.

Clinical Entrepreneurship vs. Hustle Culture

This is not about working more.

True NP entrepreneurship is not built on exhaustion. It is built on **leverage**—using expertise, experience, and insight in ways that are not limited to one-to-one visits.

If a side project:

- Requires constant urgency
- Steals recovery time
- Adds stress without meaning
- Feels performative or disconnected from your values

It is not alignment.

It is just another drain.

Aligned growth should feel **expansive**, not frantic.

Regulatory Reality (Know Before You Build)

Entrepreneurship in healthcare exists within real constraints.

Before pursuing independent ventures, NPs must understand:

- State scope-of-practice laws
- Prescriptive authority limits
- Business ownership rules
- Insurance and credentialing requirements
- Malpractice implications
- Employment contract restrictions (non-competes, moonlighting clauses)

This is not discouragement.

It is **professional maturity**.

The most successful NP entrepreneurs are cautious, informed, and patient. They build slowly—and last.

Leadership as Entrepreneurship

Not all NPs want to own businesses. Many find expansion through **leadership**.

Leadership roles allow NPs to:

- Shape systems instead of navigating broken ones
- Advocate for practice standards
- Improve workflows
- Influence policy

- Mentor future clinicians
- Protect patient safety at scale

Leadership is entrepreneurship inside institutions.

You are still creating value—just within a shared structure.

The Portfolio Career Model

One of the most sustainable long-term paths for NPs is the **portfolio career**.

Instead of one role doing everything, work is distributed:

- Clinical care (part-time or focused)
- Teaching or mentoring
- Consulting or advising
- Writing or speaking
- Leadership or program development

No single role carries the full emotional, financial, or identity load.

This model reduces burnout not by escaping care—but by **right-sizing it**.

Redefining Success Over Time

Early success feels like competence.

Mid-career success feels like balance.

Late-career success feels like contribution without depletion.

Long-term growth asks different questions:

- Can I still do this with integrity?
- Does this work leave me enough for my life?
- Am I growing—or just enduring?
- What do I want my influence to look like now?

The answers will change.

Your career should be allowed to change with them.

The Alignment Test for Growth

Before pursuing any long-term opportunity—clinical, leadership, or entrepreneurial—ask:

- Does this expand or compress my energy?
- Does it align with my current season of life?
- Does it build skills that compound?
- Does it protect my future self?
- Does it let me stay human?

If the answer is no, pause.

Growth that costs your wholeness is not growth.

It is erosion.

Final Reflection

Nurse Practitioners are trained to think long-term for patients.

This chapter asks you to apply that same wisdom to yourself.

You are not meant to practice the same way forever.

You are meant to **evolve with intention**.

The most fulfilled NPs are not those who endure the longest.

They are the ones who design careers spacious enough to grow, bend, and breathe.

Longevity is not luck.

It is alignment, practiced over time.

Chapter 40
Next Moves™ — Not Every Pivot Is an Exit

Careers rarely move in straight lines, especially in healthcare.

Next Moves™ exists to challenge one of the most persistent myths clinicians carry: that leaving a role means failure, and that staying put—no matter the cost—means resilience. In reality, career sustainability often depends on your ability to adjust course without burning everything behind you.

A pivot is not the same thing as quitting.

And staying is not always the same thing as succeeding.

Why Pivots Carry So Much Emotional Weight

Healthcare training rewards endurance. You are taught to push through discomfort, absorb pressure, and keep going. That mindset builds competence—but it can also make reassessment feel disloyal or weak.

Many clinicians delay making changes not because they lack options, but because they fear what a change might say about them.

Next Moves™ reframes pivots as *informed responses* to new information. As your understanding deepens—about the role, the system, and yourself—it is reasonable for your direction to change.

That is not instability.

It is adaptation.

Recognizing When a Role No Longer Fits

Misalignment rarely announces itself dramatically. More often, it shows up as:

- Persistent fatigue that does not improve with time
- Cognitive overload that lingers after work
- Diminishing recovery between shifts
- A sense of carrying weight that does not lift

These signals do not automatically mean you should leave. They do mean it is time to evaluate whether the mismatch is situational, structural, or personal.

Next Moves™ helps you slow down long enough to tell the difference.

Types of Pivots That Preserve Momentum

Not every pivot involves leaving clinical practice or starting over. Many adjustments preserve continuity while improving fit.

Common pivots include:

- Changing settings (inpatient to outpatient, hospital to clinic)

- Adjusting schedules or call structures
- Shifting patient populations
- Reducing scope temporarily to regain balance
- Moving into hybrid roles that combine clinical and non-clinical work

These moves often restore sustainability without discarding your training or identity.

When Leaving Is the Right Move

Sometimes, the most responsible decision is to exit a role—or even a path—that no longer aligns.

Leaving does not erase what you have learned. It does not invalidate your effort. It means you are responding to evidence rather than inertia.

Next Moves™ treats exits as one option among many, not as the default or the taboo. The goal is not to stay at all costs. The goal is to protect long-term viability.

Planning Forward Without Panic

Career decisions feel heavier when made under pressure. Next Moves™ encourages proactive planning before urgency sets in.

Ask yourself:

- What skills am I building that transfer?
- What constraints matter most right now?
- What would "better" look like—not perfect, just better?

Small, intentional moves made early often prevent forced decisions later.

The Purpose of Next Moves™

This section exists to normalize reassessment.

Healthcare careers are long. You are allowed to change within them.

A pivot is not a retreat.

It is often the most strategic way forward.

Next up: Before You Commit™ — What People Wish They Had Known Before Applying to School

Chapter 41

Before You Commit™ — What People Wish They Had Known Before Applying to School

Most regret in healthcare does not come from choosing the "wrong" role.

It comes from committing before understanding the cost.

Before You Commit™ exists for the moment *before* momentum becomes obligation—before applications are submitted, before loans are signed, before identity begins to harden around a path that feels increasingly difficult to step away from.

This section is not meant to discourage you. It is meant to surface the questions people often ask *after* the decision has already been made.

Education Is a Doorway, Not a Destination

Graduate education is frequently framed as a necessary sacrifice on the way to a better role. What is discussed less often is how that sacrifice shapes flexibility long after graduation.

Before you apply, understand:

- The full cost of attendance, not just tuition
- How long repayment realistically takes
- What income looks like in your region after graduation
- Whether projected earnings justify the debt for *you*, not in theory

Education expands opportunity—but it also narrows options if the financial burden is underestimated.

Debt Changes the Way Choices Feel

Student loans do more than affect monthly budgets. They influence tolerance.

Debt can make it harder to:

- Walk away from misaligned roles
- Reduce hours when needed
- Take lower-paying roles that might offer better support
- Pause or pivot without anxiety

Many clinicians wish they had modeled worst-case scenarios, not best-case ones. Before You Commit™ encourages you to ask what happens if compensation plateaus, if workload increases, or if your priorities change.

The Role Feels Different Once the Title Is Real

Training often emphasizes capability. Practice emphasizes responsibility.

Several clinicians report that the emotional weight of the Nurse Practitioner role felt manageable in school and overwhelming in practice—not because they lacked skill, but because decision ownership is different when there is no buffer.

Before committing to education, ask yourself:

- How do I recover from cognitive load?
- Do I prefer shared decision-making or individual accountability?
- How much uncertainty can I carry without rumination?

These questions matter more than GPA or test scores.

School Does Not Prepare You for Everything

Graduate programs prepare you to practice safely. They do not always prepare you for:

- Productivity pressure
- Documentation volume
- Negotiation
- Boundary-setting
- Organizational politics

That gap is not a failure of education. It is a reality of systems. Knowing it ahead of time helps you seek mentorship and support early.

Timing Matters More Than Urgency

One of the most common regrets is not waiting—not because waiting would have changed the decision, but because it would have clarified it.

There is no penalty for taking time to:

- Work in the field longer
- Explore adjacent roles
- Save money
- Observe the role more closely

Rushing rarely improves fit.

What People Wish They Had Asked

Looking back, many clinicians say they wish they had asked:

- What does a sustainable week actually look like?
- How often do people leave this role—and why?
- What support exists when I am uncertain?
- How does this role affect life outside of work?

Before You Commit™ exists to make those questions visible while you still have room to respond to the answers.

Why This Section Comes Last

This section is placed near the end of the book intentionally.

By now, you have seen the emotional toll, the lived workdays, the decision framework, the job market, the financial tradeoffs, and the ways careers evolve. You are no longer deciding in the abstract.

Before You Commit™ is here to help you decide with eyes open.

Whatever you choose next—yes, no, or not yet—should be a decision you can stand behind over time.

Next up: Glossary

Chapter 42

Professional Development Roadmap

Professional Development Roadmap: Planning Your NP Career Trajectory

Here's something nobody tells you when you graduate from NP school: becoming a nurse practitioner isn't the end of your professional development journey — it's the beginning. Your first day as a practicing NP marks the start of a career that will evolve dramatically over decades. The choices you make about fellowships, certifications, professional involvement, and continuing education will shape your expertise, earning potential, and career satisfaction.

This chapter is your roadmap from nervous new grad to confident expert to potential leader in your field. We'll talk about what to expect in year one versus year five versus year ten; fellowship opportunities that can accelerate your development; the certification renewal process nobody warns you about; adding specialty certifications to expand your practice; getting real value from professional organizations; and networking strategies that actually work.

Let's map out your professional development trajectory so you can be intentional about building the career you want.

What to Expect: Year 1, Year 5, and Year 10

Your first year as an NP looks nothing like your fifth year, which looks nothing like your tenth. Understanding the typical progression helps you set realistic expectations and plan strategically.

Year One: Survival Mode and Skill Building

Your first year as an NP is intense. You have the knowledge and the license, but not yet the experience or pattern recognition that comes with time. Everything takes longer. You second-guess yourself constantly. You look things up multiple times a day. You worry about missing something important.

This is completely normal.

In year one, your priorities are simple and critical:

- Build clinical confidence
- Develop efficient workflows
- Establish safe, sustainable habits

You're not trying to be the "best NP" in your organization. You're trying to be competent, safe, and steadily improving. Seek out opportunities to see a wide variety of conditions. Take complex patients when you have support. Ask questions — even when you feel like you "should" already know the answer.

Your documentation will likely take forever. You may stay late most days finishing charts. Your templates aren't optimized yet. You're still learning your EHR. All of this improves with time. By month six, you'll be noticeably faster. By month twelve, you'll feel like a different provider than you were on day one.

Financially, year one is about stabilizing:

- Start repaying student loans
- Build a basic emergency fund
- Capture any employer retirement match

You don't have to max out retirement accounts, buy a house, and become debt-free in your first year. Make progress, not perfection.

Professionally, join at least one professional organization in year one. A national membership (like AANP) and your state NP association will give you education, advocacy, and networking you simply can't get alone. Budget a few hundred dollars annually for memberships.

Year one is also when you should seriously consider whether fellowship training interests you (more on that later). Many programs recruit during your final NP year or soon after graduation — so don't wait if it's on your radar.

Year Five: Finding Your Stride

By year five, you're a different clinician.

You've seen enough patients that pattern recognition kicks in. You can spot a sick patient from across the room. You're no longer just following algorithms — you're integrating them with your own growing clinical judgment. Documentation is faster. You know your scope, your limits, and when to consult or refer.

Year five is when many NPs start to feel restless. You've mastered the basics and you're ready for new challenges. This is a natural pivot point.

Common year-five moves include:

- Adding specialty certifications
- Moving into leadership, education, or advanced clinical roles
- Switching specialties or settings
- Taking on precepting and mentorship

Financially, year five often brings more stability:

- Debt is reduced or significantly managed
- Emergency savings are in place
- Retirement contributions are increasing
- You may be considering home ownership if you haven't already

Professionally, year five is when you start giving back. Consider:

- Precepting students
- Presenting at local or state conferences
- Serving on committees or task forces

This is also a great time to add specialty certifications. With five years behind you, you have enough experience to pursue advanced credentials and enough career ahead to benefit from them.

Year Ten: Expert and Leader

By year ten, you're a seasoned expert.

You're the person others come to for help with tricky cases. You've managed complications, odd presentations, and everything in between. Your clinical judgment is refined. You can handle complexity and acuity with confidence.

Around this time, many NPs pivot into:

• Clinical leadership roles (lead NP, clinical director)

• Education (faculty, preceptor coordinators)

• Policy and advocacy work

• Highly specialized clinical or consultant roles

Not everyone wants formal leadership or administrative roles — and that's okay. Many NPs choose to remain primarily clinical, deepening their expertise while staying at the bedside or clinic. Both paths are valuable. What matters is choosing intentionally rather than drifting.

Financially, year ten often brings:

• Peak or near-peak earning potential for your specialty and region

• A solid understanding of compensation models (including RVUs, if relevant)

• Mature retirement accounts and clearer long-term financial goals

Professionally, you're established. You have a reputation, a network, and clarity about what kind of practice is sustainable for you.

Timelines vary. Some NPs feel like experts by year seven; others take fifteen years to feel fully confident. Your setting matters too — year five in a high-volume urban ER is different from year five in a rural family practice. Treat these timelines as general guideposts, not rigid rules.

Fellowship Opportunities: Accelerated Learning for New Grads

NP fellowships are structured postgraduate training programs (typically 6–12 months) that provide mentored clinical experience in a specific specialty. They're similar in concept to physician residencies, but shorter and not required for practice.

What Fellowships Offer

Fellowships provide:

- Intensive clinical training in a focused area
- Close preceptorship and feedback
- Reduced patient volumes while you learn
- Regular didactic or seminar time
- Exposure to complex cases earlier in your career

You graduate with advanced skills, stronger confidence, and a clear specialty focus. This often gives you a competitive edge for specialty positions.

Some fellowships:

- Are paid (usually at a lower salary than a standard NP role)
- Offer benefits such as health insurance or loan assistance

Many graduates report feeling better prepared for independent practice than peers who entered the workforce directly.

Common Fellowship Focus Areas

- Hospital medicine / inpatient care
- Emergency medicine
- Critical care / ICU
- Cardiology
- Orthopedics
- Pain management
- Palliative care
- Women's health
- Primary care in underserved settings

The Application Process

Most fellowships recruit during your final NP year or immediately afterward. Expect:

- CV
- Personal statement
- Letters of recommendation
- Interviews

These programs can be competitive, so:

• Research options early (ideally by your penultimate semester)

• Track deadlines (often November–January for summer starts)

• Talk to current or former fellows when possible

Missing deadlines usually means waiting another year.

Financial Considerations

Paid fellowships often offer salaries in the $50,000–$70,000 range, usually lower than standard NP roles. Unpaid fellowships may require outside work or savings to support yourself.

Think in terms of return on investment. If a year-long fellowship leads to higher-paying roles, specialty opportunities, or faster confidence in a complex field, it can pay off financially and professionally over time.

Is Fellowship Right for You?

Fellowships may be a good fit if:

• You want to enter a highly specialized or acute setting

• You thrive with structured mentorship

• You can temporarily accept lower income

• You're changing into a new specialty and want formal training

They may be less necessary if:

- You're entering a supportive primary care role with strong onboarding
- You need to maximize income immediately
- You already have substantial experience as an RN in the same specialty

Many excellent NPs never do fellowships and grow through on-the-job mentorship. Fellowships are an accelerator, not a requirement.

Board Certification Renewal: The Process Nobody Warns You About

Passing your certification exam is a huge milestone — but it's not a one-and-done event. Your NP certification expires (usually in five years), and you must renew it to maintain your ability to practice.

The Basics

- Certification typically lasts **five years** from your exam date.
- Renewal requires:
  - Continuing education (CE) hours
  - Practice hours (for many certifying bodies)
  - Renewal fees

You are responsible for tracking your expiration date. Do not rely solely on reminder emails.

Continuing Education Requirements

Most NP certifications require **75–100 contact hours** of CE over five years, with a set number of pharmacology hours.

Practical tips:

- Start earning and tracking hours in year one, not year four.
- Keep all CE certificates in a dedicated folder (physical or digital).
- Use conferences, online modules, and employer- provided education to meet requirements.
- Choose CE that actually strengthens your practice, not just "check-the-box" content.

Practice Hour Requirements

Many certifying bodies require proof of a minimum number of NP practice hours (often around 1,000 over five years). This is usually simple if you work consistently.

If you:

- Take extended leave
- Change specialties
- Work in an area that doesn't obviously match your certification

...check your certifying body's exact rules and plan ahead.

Fees, Timeline, and Avoiding Panic

- Renewal fees typically run **$200–$400**.
- Some employers reimburse renewal costs — ask about this benefit.
- You can usually begin renewing up to a year before expiration.

Begin the process at least **three months** before your deadline. Waiting until the last minute is a recipe for stress.

If you let your certification lapse, you may:

- Be unable to practice
- Owe additional fees
- In some cases, need to retake the exam

All of that is avoidable with planning.

Adding Specialty Certifications: Expanding Your Scope and Marketability

Your primary NP certification defines your population focus (FNP, AGNP, etc.), but specialty certifications can highlight advanced expertise and open new doors.

Why Add Specialty Certifications?

Specialty certifications can:

- Differentiate you in a crowded job market
- Signal advanced knowledge in a focused area
- Qualify you for specialized roles or clinics
- Sometimes support higher compensation or unique billing opportunities

They can also keep your career interesting and aligned with evolving interests.

Common Specialty Certifications for NPs

Examples include:

- **Diabetes care and education**
- **Obesity / weight management**
- **Dermatology practice**
- **Hospice and palliative care**
- **Emergency or critical care specialties**
- **Wound care, pain management, HIV care, oncology**, and others

Each certification has its own:

- Practice hour requirements
- CE requirements
- Exam
- Fees

The Process and Timing

Before pursuing a specialty certification:

- Confirm eligibility requirements (practice hours, CE, degree level)
- Budget for exam and prep costs
- Plan study time

Timing matters. Don't stack a specialty exam on top of your first NP job transition or during a period of major personal stress. Give yourself enough experience in the specialty to make the exam meaningful and manageable.

Maintaining Multiple Certifications

Each certification adds:

- Renewal fees
- CE requirements
- Tracking and documentation

Be realistic. It's better to maintain one or two certifications you actively use than collect credentials you don't keep up or don't use in practice.

Professional Organization Membership: Getting Real Value

Every NP should belong to at least one professional organization — but many pay dues without using the benefits. Let's fix that.

Which Organizations to Join

At minimum, consider:

- **A national NP organization** (e.g., AANP)
- **Your state NP association**

Later, you might add:

- **Specialty organizations** related to your practice area

You don't need to join everything at once. Start with the two that give you the broadest advocacy and education, then add others as your career focus sharpens.

Using Your Memberships Wisely

Get your money's worth by:

- Using member discounts for CE and conferences

- Reading member journals or newsletters regularly
- Accessing practice resources and toolkits
- Staying updated on policy changes affecting NPs
- Using directories or forums for clinical and career questions

Getting Involved (Without Overcommitting)

Deeper involvement can include:

- Serving on committees
- Presenting at conferences
- Writing for newsletters or blogs
- Serving on the board at the state or local level

These roles expand your network, build leadership skills, and strengthen your CV.

If you've paid dues for years and never used benefits, reassess. It's okay to prioritize one or two high-value memberships rather than scattering your resources.

Conferences and Networking: Building Relationships and Expertise

Conferences offer education **and** connection — and both matter.

Choosing Conferences Strategically

Options include:

- **National NP conferences** — broad content and a big-picture view

- **State or regional conferences** — local networking and policy updates

- **Specialty conferences** — deep dives into your area of focus

Consider:

- Your learning needs

- Your budget

- Employer support or CE budget

A well-chosen conference can provide most of your CE for the year plus important networking opportunities.

Getting Maximum Value

To make conferences count:

- Engage in sessions — ask questions, take notes, think about application to your practice.

- Talk to people — at meals, between sessions, in the exhibit hall.

- Visit the exhibit hall with curiosity, not just a swag bag.

- Follow up with people you meet via email or LinkedIn afterward.

Networking Strategies That Actually Work

Networking is simply relationship-building with a professional purpose.

Principles for Authentic Networking

- Be curious, not salesy. Ask about others' roles, settings, and paths.

• Offer value when you can — share a resource, make an introduction, answer a question.

• Maintain your connections — occasional check-ins keep relationships alive.

• Use LinkedIn as a professional home base for your network.

Networking is not about collecting business cards. It's about building a web of people you can learn from and collaborate with — and who can do the same with you.

If You're Introverted

You don't have to "work the room." Instead:

• Aim for a few meaningful one-on-one conversations

• Use online communities and LinkedIn

• Give yourself breaks at in-person events

• Focus on depth over breadth

Introverts are often excellent networkers because they listen well and build strong, lasting relationships.

Your Professional Development Action Plan

Professional development is a lifelong journey, not a checklist. Here's a framework you can adapt:

Year One

• Focus on clinical competence and safe practice

• Establish documentation and workflow habits

• Join at least one national and one state NP organization

- Explore fellowship options if they align with your goals

Years Two to Five

- Consider specialty certifications that match your interests and practice
- Begin presenting, writing, or precepting
- Attend at least one conference each year
- Refine your financial plan as your income stabilizes

Years Five to Ten

- Explore leadership, education, or advanced specialty roles if desired
- Deepen involvement in organizations (committees, boards, policy work)
- Build your professional reputation through presentations, publications, or projects

Throughout Your Career

- Maintain certification and CE requirements
- Stay current with clinical guidelines and health policy
- Revisit your career goals every few years
- Maintain and grow your professional network

Keep a professional portfolio that includes:

- Certifications and licenses
- CE records
- Presentations and publications

- Committees and leadership roles
- Awards and recognitions

This makes updating your CV, renewing certifications, or applying for new roles much easier.

Set an **annual professional development budget and plan.** Decide in advance:

- Which conferences you'll attend
- Which memberships you'll maintain
- Which certifications you'll pursue or renew

You are your own most important professional asset. The time, money, and energy you invest in your growth as an NP will pay off in confidence, opportunity, and satisfaction.

The most fulfilled NPs are not necessarily the ones with the most credentials — they're the ones who shape their careers intentionally. They choose fellowships, certifications, organizations, and relationships that align with the kind of work and life they actually want.

You've done the hard work to become an NP. Now, this roadmap is here to help you become the NP you're meant to be.

Chapter 43

Technology and Innovation

Technology and Innovation: Navigating the Digital Transformation of Healthcare

Here's the uncomfortable truth: technology can either make your life as an NP dramatically easier or turn your workday into a frustrating marathon of clicking through endless screens. The difference comes down to knowing which tools actually help, how to use them efficiently, and what red flags to watch for when evaluating digital systems.

This chapter isn't about becoming a tech expert. It's about practical knowledge that allows you to work smarter, deliver better care, and avoid the digital burnout that's becoming increasingly common in healthcare. We'll look at electronic health records, telehealth regulations, artificial intelligence, patient communication platforms, and the digital tools reshaping the NP role.

Let's cut through the marketing hype and focus on what truly matters.

Electronic Health Records: The Good, the Bad, and the Epic

Whether you love them or hate them, EHRs are the backbone of modern clinical practice. You'll spend a significant portion of your day interacting with your EHR, so understanding the major systems—and how to work efficiently within them—is essential.

The Major Players

Epic

Epic is the giant of the EHR world and widely used in large hospital systems and academic medical centers. It's powerful, fully integrated, and capable of handling everything from documentation to order entry to messaging. The downside is its steep learning curve. New users often feel overwhelmed by the menus, shortcuts, and workflow options. Once you master it, however, Epic becomes highly efficient. Invest early in customizing templates, learning dotphrases, and asking experienced colleagues for tips.

Cerner

Cerner is another major system, especially in hospital settings. It excels in inpatient workflows but can feel clunky in outpatient environments. Its interface style differs from Epic's, so some clinicians love it while others struggle. Like Epic, Cerner requires time and training to master.

Athenahealth

Athenahealth is popular in ambulatory settings and private practices. It's cloud-based, intuitive, and integrates practice management functions with clinical documentation. While it may not have the advanced specialty features of Epic or Cerner, it's user-friendly and efficient for outpatient workflows.

eClinicalWorks, NextGen, Allscripts

These appear frequently in small to mid-sized practices. Each has strengths—eCW for customization, NextGen for billing integration, Allscripts for flexibility across settings.

Evaluating an EHR During Your Job Search

Ask:

- Which EHR does the practice use?
- How long has it been implemented?
- What training is provided?
- Can you shadow a clinician using it?

Pay attention to how staff talk about the EHR. Constant complaints often signal poor implementation or unrealistic documentation expectations—not necessarily a bad system.

Also ask about IT support: when something breaks, who helps you, and how quickly?

Documentation Strategies for Efficiency

EHR time is one of the biggest drivers of NP burnout. To work efficiently:

- **Master templates and shortcuts.** Invest early in building templates for common visits.
- **Document during or immediately after the visit.** Delayed documentation equals staying late.

• **Use voice recognition or scribes when available.** These can be game-changing.

• **Avoid over-documenting.** Include what's clinically relevant and required for billing—nothing more.

• **Close notes promptly.** Aim to finish before leaving for the day.

Interoperability Challenges

Different EHRs still struggle to communicate, which means outside records often arrive via faxed PDFs. Ask if your employer participates in a **Health Information Exchange (HIE)** or uses tools like Epic's **Care Everywhere**, which allow seamless record sharing.

Telehealth: A New Frontier That's Here to Stay

Telehealth surged during the pandemic and will remain a core part of care delivery. NPs must understand best practices, legal requirements, and how to maintain care quality virtually.

Telehealth Modalities

• **Synchronous video visits**

• **Asynchronous store-and-forward** (common in dermatology)

• **Remote patient monitoring** (RPM)

• **Telephone-only visits** (still widely used)

Best Practices for Telehealth Visits

• Choose a quiet, professional setting with good lighting.

• Look at the camera to simulate eye contact.

• Adapt your exam: observe, instruct, and use patient-provided data.

• Know when telehealth isn't enough and transition to in-person care.

• Document modality, patient location, and participants.

Licensure and Legal Considerations

You must be licensed in the **state where the patient physically is** during the visit.

Interstate NP compacts are still limited, so verify state rules before practicing cross-state telehealth.

Reimbursement and Prescribing

Telehealth reimbursement remains strong—though evolving. Use correct telehealth codes and modifiers. Controlled substances often require an initial in-person visit. Policies change frequently; stay current with state and federal updates.

Artificial Intelligence and Clinical Decision Support

AI is increasingly integrated into everyday workflows. Used correctly, it enhances safety and efficiency—but it never replaces clinical judgment.

What AI Can Do

• Flag drug interactions and contraindications

• Assist in diagnostic interpretation (imaging, ECGs, dermatology)

• Generate draft clinical notes

• Identify patients at high risk for complications

- Analyze large datasets for patterns clinicians might miss

What AI Cannot Do

- Replace your clinical reasoning
- Understand patient context or preferences
- Navigate ethical complexity
- Perform well outside the populations it was trained on

Using AI Responsibly

- Verify AI-generated suggestions
- Know tool limits
- Be transparent with patients when AI assists in care
- Stay informed as tools evolve rapidly

Patient Portals and Digital Communication

Patient portals are now standard, but they also create new workloads.

Managing the Portal Inbox

- Set clear response-time expectations.
- Delegate administrative messages to staff.
- Redirect urgent or complex issues to phone or visits.
- Track portal time if your contract addresses it.

Effective Portal Messaging

- Be concise and jargon-free.
- Document clinically relevant exchanges.

- Convert prolonged message threads into visits.
- Use templates for frequently asked questions.

Remote Patient Monitoring: The Future of Chronic Care

RPM uses connected devices to transmit patient data directly to clinicians.

How RPM Works

Patients use devices such as BP cuffs, glucometers, scales, or pulse oximeters that send readings automatically. Abnormal values prompt early intervention—often preventing hospitalizations.

Implementing RPM

- Select appropriate patients.
- Choose accurate, user-friendly devices.
- Establish clear monitoring workflows.
- Understand billing requirements.
- Prioritize patient engagement.

Common RPM Devices

- BP monitors for hypertension
- CGMs for diabetes
- Pulse oximeters for COPD and HF
- Scales for HF
- Wearables for rhythm or activity monitoring

Digital Prescribing: Beyond Basic E-Prescribing

Modern platforms support:

- **Electronic prescribing (EPCS for controlled substances)**
- **Prior authorization automation**
- **Medication cost transparency**
- **Pharmacogenomics integration**
- **Specialty pharmacy coordination**

These tools improve safety, adherence, and efficiency—when used correctly.

Staying Current Without Burning Out

Technology evolves constantly. To stay grounded:

- Follow professional organizations.
- Participate in tech committees or pilot programs.
- Learn from colleagues.
- Advocate for clinician-friendly technology.
- Set boundaries for digital communication.

Your Technology Action Plan

- Ask detailed questions about technology during your job search.
- Invest time early to learn new systems.
- Build efficient documentation habits immediately.
- Establish and maintain communication boundaries.

- Adopt tools that genuinely solve problems—not every shiny new product.
- Speak up when technology hinders care.

Final Thought

The digital transformation of healthcare is ongoing. NPs who thrive aren't the most tech-savvy—they're the ones who approach technology thoughtfully, using it as a tool to elevate care rather than letting it dominate their practice. You don't need to be an expert, but you do need to be a **savvy user**. This chapter gives you everything you need to step confidently into that role.

Chapter 44
Side Hustles

Side Hustles for the Modern Nurse Practitioner

More Ways to Practice Your Purpose

Healthcare has never been one-directional, and neither are Nurse Practitioners. Clinical care is your foundation, but it doesn't have to be your ceiling. Whether you're craving extra income, creative expression, schedule flexibility, or a stepping-stone into new professional territory, side hustles let you explore dimensions of your career that your 9-to-5 rarely reveals.

This chapter is your guide to seven high-impact NP-friendly side hustles — each one proven, accessible, and aligned with the skills you already use every day. These aren't fantasies. They are real, revenue-generating pathways NPs are walking right now.

Telehealth Consulting

Care with a passport.

Telehealth lets you practice across state lines (with proper licensure/collaborative agreements), work from your couch, and customize your hours. Brands, startups, urgent care platforms, and chronic-care companies rely on NPs to deliver fast, accurate virtual care.

What You Do:

- Evaluate acute or chronic conditions via video

- Provide medication management

- Write protocols or triage workflows

- Offer asynchronous consults for patients or partner clinicians

Why It Works:

- Flexible hours (pick up 1–10 hours/week)

- Growing market

- Requires minimal setup

Earning Potential:

$40–$100/hour depending on platform and specialty.

Expert Witness Work

Your charting skills, but paid like a lawyer.

Attorneys hire Nurse Practitioners as medical experts to review records, decode standards of care, and testify. If you have a specialty or years of clinical experience, this can be an extremely lucrative niche.

What You Do:

- Review medical records for plaintiff or defense
- Explain standards of care
- Provide written opinions
- Testify in depositions or court

Why It Works:

- High hourly rates
- Uses skills you already have
- No patient care required

Earning Potential:

$150–$600/hour for reviews; $2,000–$5,000/day for testimony.

Medical Writing

Your clinical brain + your storyteller voice.

Healthcare companies, publishers, journals, startups, and continuing-education groups need clinicians who can translate medicine into clear, trustworthy content. NPs make outstanding medical writers because you already simplify complex ideas for patients every day.

What You Do:

- Write patient education materials
- Draft clinical guides, CE modules, or protocols
- Author articles for health media
- Contribute to textbooks or digital platforms

Why It Works:

- Creative

- Remote

- Excellent portfolio builder

- Scales into books, courses, brand partnerships

Earning Potential:

$0.20–$1.00 per word, or $50–$150/hour.

Healthcare Education & Training

Teach what you know, shape who they become.

From nursing schools to online academies, simulation labs, and corporate wellness programs — educators with real-world clinical experience are in high demand.

What You Do:

- Teach clinical skills or specialty modules

- Serve as a guest lecturer

- Run workshops on communication, documentation, or procedures

- Develop CEU courses

Why It Works:

- Aligned with NP leadership roles

- Expands your professional network

- Provides recurring income

Earning Potential:

$300–$1,000 per lecture; $1,000–$5,000 per CE course.

Product Development Consulting

Help shape the tools clinicians actually use.

Companies building stethoscopes, EMRs, AI triage tools, medical devices, patient-monitoring systems, and wellness apps desperately need clinician input. NPs offer frontline insight that engineers and designers can't replicate.

What You Do:

- Test prototypes

- Advise on workflow, usability, and patient safety

- Participate in product development meetings

- Co-create clinical tools or content

Why It Works:

- Your clinical perspective is rare and valuable

- Opportunity for royalties or equity

- Great for NPs who like innovation

Earning Potential:

$75–$200/hour; equity or royalties possible.

Clinical Research

Be the bridge between science and care.

Research organizations and pharma sponsors need NPs to help evaluate safety, efficacy, and patient response. If you enjoy evidence-based practice, this is a natural extension of your NP brain.

What You Do:

- Conduct study visits
- Collect data and perform assessments
- Review protocols
- Serve as a sub-investigator

Why It Works:

- Work can be per-diem or project-based
- Elevates your clinical credibility
- Excellent for NPs interested in academia or industry roles

Earning Potential:

$50–$100/hour; higher for specialty trials.

Health Coaching

When patients need more than a prescription.

As an NP, you understand behavior change, barriers, and the emotional landscape of wellness. Health coaching lets you guide clients toward lifestyle transformation through individualized support.

What You Do:

- Assess lifestyle, sleep, nutrition, stress, movement
- Build weekly action plans
- Provide ongoing accountability via video or messaging

- Offer specialty coaching (diabetes, women's health, cardiac, etc.)

Why It Works:

- Extremely flexible

- Cash-pay

- High impact and relationship-centered

- Can evolve into group coaching or online programs

Earning Potential:

$75–$200/session; $500–$2,500 per multi-week coaching program.

Bringing It All Together

Side hustles are not random—they're intentional extensions of the NP identity.

Some fuel your creativity.

Some expand your influence.

Some strengthen your financial well-being.

And some — if aligned — open doors you never knew existed.

Your NP license isn't just a credential.

It's a compass.

And every side hustle in this chapter gives you another way to follow it.

Chapter 45

Full-Reduced-Restricted Practice

- **Full Practice**

State law allows NPs to independently evaluate, diagnose, order/interpret tests, and prescribe (including controlled substances) under the exclusive authority of the board of nursing, with no permanent requirement for physician collaboration or supervision.

- **Reduced Practice**

The NP's ability to practice and/or prescribe is limited in at least one element (often prescribing or practice ownership). A career-long collaborative agreement with a physician or other specified provider is required *or* state law restricts certain settings or medications.

- **Restricted Practice**

State law requires career-long physician supervision, delegation, or team management for diagnosis, treatment, and prescribing. NPs cannot function as fully independent prescribers and typically must work under a supervisory agreement.

Quick-Reference Table: NP Practice Authority by State (2025)

Suggested heading in book:

State-by-State Nurse Practitioner Practice Authority (AANP Categories)

Current as of December, 2025 — always verify with your State Board of Nursing before making career or relocation decisions.

State

NP Practice Authority Category*

Alabama

Reduced Practice

Alaska

Full Practice

Arizona

Full Practice

Arkansas

Reduced Practice

California

Restricted Practice

Colorado

Full Practice

Connecticut

Full Practice

Delaware

Full Practice

Florida

Restricted Practice

Georgia

Restricted Practice

Hawaii

Full Practice

Idaho

Full Practice

Illinois

Reduced Practice

Indiana

Reduced Practice

Iowa

Full Practice

Kansas

Full Practice

Kentucky

Reduced Practice

Louisiana

Reduced Practice

Maine

Full Practice

Maryland

Full Practice

Massachusetts

Full Practice

Michigan

Restricted Practice

Minnesota

Full Practice

Mississippi

Reduced Practice

Missouri

Restricted Practice

Montana

Full Practice

Nebraska

Full Practice

Nevada

Full Practice

New Hampshire

Full Practice

New Jersey

Reduced Practice

New Mexico

Full Practice

New York

Full Practice

North Carolina

Restricted Practice

North Dakota

Full Practice

Ohio

Reduced Practice

Oklahoma

Restricted Practice

Oregon

Full Practice

Pennsylvania

Reduced Practice

Rhode Island

Full Practice

South Carolina

Restricted Practice

South Dakota

Full Practice

Tennessee

Restricted Practice

Texas

Restricted Practice

Utah

Full Practice

Vermont

Full Practice

Virginia

Restricted Practice

Washington

Full Practice

West Virginia

Reduced Practice

Wisconsin

Reduced Practice

Wyoming

Full Practice

District of Columbia

Full Practice

*Categories based on AANP's **Full / Reduced / Restricted** practice environment model, as summarized in 2025 national reference tables.

- **Full Practice Territories:** Guam, Northern Mariana Islands

- **Reduced Practice Territories:** American Samoa, Puerto Rico, U.S. Virgin Islands

Important: Nurse practitioner practice and prescriptive authority laws change frequently. This table reflects national reference data available in 2025, but it is not legal advice and may not capture the most recent legislative updates in your state.

Before accepting a position, signing a contract, or relocating, always confirm current NP practice and prescriptive authority with your State Board of Nursing and, when needed, consult your professional association or a healthcare attorney.

Chapter 46

Alignment Check and Reflection

How to Use *The Alignment Check*

The Alignment Check — 10 Questions That Matter Most is your personal pause button. It's designed to help you translate what you've just read into something real — your own clarity, curiosity, and next steps.

Think of it as a guided mirror: instead of telling you who to be, it helps you notice what already fits and what doesn't. Use it slowly, honestly, and without judgment. There are no right answers — only revealing ones.

Before You Begin

1 Find quiet. You'll get more from this reflection if you give it space.

2 Keep a notebook or your phone nearby. Jot your thoughts without editing; the rawest notes often hold the truth.

3 Read one role at a time. Don't rush through multiple **SCRUB*fit*™** profiles. Let each one breathe.

How to Work Through the 10 Questions

- **After each profile or category,** reread *The Alignment Check* slowly, question by question.

- **Highlight what resonates.** If a question makes your heart beat faster — that's a sign of alignment. If it makes you sigh or hesitate — that's a signal, too.

- **Circle your top three responses.** These are your "alignment anchors." They point toward careers, settings, or values that match who you are.

- **Revisit the list later.** Your answers may shift as your experiences grow; alignment is a moving target, not a fixed destination.

When to Use It

- **Early exploration:** When you're still figuring out which healthcare roles fit you best.

- **Career transition:** When burnout, boredom, or curiosity says, "Maybe it's time for something different."

- **Realignment check-in:** Every six months, take five minutes to reread your answers and see what's changed.

Why It Matters

The Alignment Check helps bridge the gap between who you are and where you belong. It turns passive reading into active discovery — transforming information into insight, and insight into alignment.

The Alignment Check — 10 Questions That Matter Most

1 What first drew you to this career — curiosity, compassion, or circumstance?

2 Which part of this role feels like *you at your best*?

3 Which part would likely test your patience, endurance, or alignment?

4 How does this profession match your values, pace, and preferred kind of pressure?

5 Could you see yourself thriving in the environments where this role usually works — and why or why not?

6 What skills or experiences could you start developing right now to move closer to this path?

7 Who in your life models the professionalism or calm you'd want to bring to this career?

8 If you shadowed someone in this field for a day, what would you hope to learn about their mindset?

9 How would success in this career *feel* — not just look — in your everyday life?

10 After reading this section, does this role feel aligned, misaligned, or somewhere in between — and what does that tell you about your next step?

Chapter 47

PACES™ and CARESET™

PACES™ & CARESET™ in Nurse Practitioner Practice

Why This Career Fits Some People Beautifully — and Breaks Others Quietly

On paper, Nurse Practitioner looks like the answer.

Autonomy. Advanced clinical decision-making. Prescriptive authority. Continuity with patients. Respect. Flexibility. Impact. For many people, becoming an NP feels like finally stepping into the kind of medicine they imagined when they chose healthcare in the first place.

And yet, alongside that promise, there's a quieter reality.

Some Nurse Practitioners feel energized, stretched, and deeply aligned.

Others feel depleted, overextended, and vaguely unsettled — even when they're competent, successful, and doing everything "right."

PACES™ and CARESET™ exist to explain *why.*

Not to judge Nurse Practitioner practice — but to show how **fit** operates inside it.

Nurse Practitioner Is Not One Job

Before PACES™ or CARESET™ can make sense, one truth has to be clear:

Nurse Practitioner is not a single experience.

Family practice, acute care, specialty clinics, inpatient services, telehealth, urgent care, academic roles, leadership, and concierge medicine all carry the same title — but radically different daily realities.

Alignment isn't about whether NP is "right."

It's about **which version of NP practice fits your internal wiring and external needs.**

That's where PACES™ starts.

PACES™: How *You* Meet NP Work

Personality

Nurse Practitioner practice requires comfort with *incomplete information.* You assess, diagnose, and treat — often without the safety net of immediate oversight. Some people find that thrilling. Others find it quietly exhausting.

If your personality leans toward:

- steady confidence

- tolerance for ambiguity
- relational continuity
- measured decision-making

NP practice often feels natural.

If you require constant validation, immediate closure, or strict protocols, some NP environments may feel destabilizing — not because you're incapable, but because the *fit* is off.

Aptitude

NPs rely heavily on synthesis — pulling together symptoms, history, labs, patient behavior, and context into decisions that unfold over time.

Strong aptitude for NP practice often shows up as:

- pattern recognition
- clinical curiosity
- comfort explaining "why" to patients
- ability to hold responsibility without freezing

This is not about intelligence. It's about *how* you think.

Constraints

NP roles often blur boundaries. Charting follows you home. Patient panels grow quietly. Availability expands unless guarded intentionally.

Constraints matter here more than people admit:

- caregiving responsibilities

- physical stamina
- emotional bandwidth
- tolerance for cognitive load

PACES™ insists you name these honestly — not after burnout, but before.

Experience

Your past matters in NP practice.

Former bedside nurses may carry deep patient intuition — and also moral residue. Former paramedics may excel in decisiveness but struggle with slower continuity. New graduates may bring openness but feel overwhelmed by scope.

NP practice amplifies what you bring with you. PACES™ helps you recognize that amplification before it surprises you.

Situation

A role that fits you at 28 may not fit you at 45.

Early NP careers often involve intensity, learning curves, and proving ground environments. Later seasons may call for specialization, leadership, teaching, or reduced volume.

PACES™ normalizes evolution. It rejects the idea that changing direction means failure.

CARESET™: The Conditions That Make or Break NP Practice

If PACES™ explains *you*, CARESET™ explains *why the same NP role feels radically different in different places.*

Culture

In some organizations, NPs are trusted clinicians. In others, they're treated as cost-saving substitutes or permanently supervised trainees.

Culture determines whether your voice is welcomed or tolerated — and that distinction matters more than compensation.

Autonomy

NP autonomy varies wildly by state, organization, and specialty.

Some NPs thrive when autonomy is high. Others prefer structured collaboration. Misalignment here creates constant friction — either feeling constrained or feeling exposed.

Resources

Staffing ratios. Support staff. Appointment length. Technology. Referral access.

When resources are thin, NPs absorb the strain — often silently. CARESET™ names resource scarcity as an environmental issue, not a personal failing.

Expectations

Are you expected to:

- see more patients every quarter?
- manage increasingly complex cases without added support?

• provide emotional care without protected time?

Unspoken expectations erode alignment faster than hard work ever could.

Structure

Clinic schedules, call requirements, documentation systems, and productivity metrics all shape NP life.

Some NPs thrive in predictable structure. Others need flexibility. Structure isn't good or bad — it just has to match you.

Environment

Physical space. Noise. Pace. Emotional intensity.

An NP may love primary care but hate urgent care. Love telehealth but dread inpatient rounds. Environment matters.

Team

Team dynamics often determine whether NP practice feels collaborative or isolating.

Strong teams buffer stress. Weak teams magnify it.

CARESET™ makes this visible instead of personal.

What Alignment Actually Looks Like for NPs

When PACES™ and CARESET™ align, NP practice feels:

• demanding but sustainable

• intellectually engaging without constant depletion

- emotionally meaningful without collapse
- challenging without chronic resentment

When they don't align, the symptoms appear quietly:

- constant fatigue
- irritability that feels "out of character"
- dread without obvious cause
- questioning the profession instead of the conditions

PACES™ and CARESET™ redirect that question.

Not *"What's wrong with me?"*

But *"Which part of this isn't aligned?"*

Why This Matters More for NPs Than Most Roles

Nurse Practitioners sit at a unique intersection:

- high responsibility
- variable authority
- deep patient relationships
- expanding expectations

That combination is powerful — and dangerous without alignment.

PACES™ & CARESET™ don't protect you from hard days.

They protect you from *misplaced endurance*.

They give you permission to adjust:

- setting instead of specialty
- environment instead of profession
- structure instead of identity

Reading the Rest of This ScrubTale™

As you move through the Day-in-the-Life chapters, career maps, financial realities, and reflections ahead, use PACES™ and CARESET™ as quiet companions.

Notice:

- where you lean in
- where you tense up
- where you feel seen
- where you feel resistant

Those reactions are data.

Alignment isn't about choosing the "best" path.

It's about choosing the path that lets you stay whole.

And Nurse Practitioner practice, when aligned, can be one of the most sustaining, meaningful, and impactful roles in healthcare.

Not because it's easy.

But because it fits.

Chapter 48
Pros and Cons

Is the Nurse Practitioner Path Right for You?

The Pros, the Cons, and the Truth in Between

Becoming a Nurse Practitioner isn't just choosing a career — it's choosing a *way of moving through the world.* A way of thinking, seeing, caring, deciding, advocating, interpreting, balancing, and stitching together the science of medicine with the humanity of nursing.

Some people hear that and feel a spark.

Others feel a warning bell.

Both reactions matter — both are data.

If you're reading this book, you're already in motion. You're not just curious; you're discerning. You're evaluating alignment — that invisible force that determines whether you thrive, stagnate, or burn out. So before we walk into clinical rooms and day-in-the-life chapters, let's pause and look honestly at the life you're considering.

Let's talk about the **real** pros, the **real** cons, and the **real** questions that separate "I think I want this" from "I am made for this."

The Pros — What Makes This Path Worth It

1. You get to make decisions that change lives.

NPs don't just "support care."

They *deliver* it.

From diagnosing pneumonia to managing diabetes to recognizing when something is far more serious — your clinical judgment becomes the pivot point in someone's story.

That weight? It's not a burden.

For the right person, it's a privilege.

2. Autonomy with scaffolding.

Depending on your state, setting, and certification, you may practice independently or collaboratively — but either way, you're trusted as a primary clinical decision-maker. You'll manage panels, lead visits, and shape care plans with a level of autonomy rare in healthcare.

You're not "helping the doctor."

You *are* the provider.

3. The flexibility is unmatched.

NPs pivot.

From family practice to cardiology.

From inpatient to outpatient.

From community clinics to telehealth hubs.

If you crave variety, evolution, and the ability to reinvent your career without starting from scratch, the NP path is one of the most flexible roles in modern medicine.

4. Deep, relationship-centered care.

You get time — not unlimited time, not perfect time, but more time than many healthcare roles allow — to listen, teach, coach, and genuinely connect.

NPs are often the providers patients trust the most.

The ones they request by name.

The ones they remember.

That has power.

5. A leadership role that doesn't require stepping away from patients.

You can lead hospitals, clinics, initiatives, teams — all while still keeping your hands on the work. You don't have to choose leadership *or* patient care. You can weave both.

6. Purpose you can feel in your bones.

There is a moment every NP knows:

You catch something early.

You reassure someone who is terrified.

You sit with a patient in the doorway of a diagnosis.

You make a call that matters.

That moment imprints on you.

It becomes your reminder that this path is sacred work.

The Cons — The Parts No One Tells You Early Enough

1. The emotional load is heavy.

You will celebrate victories — and you will carry losses.

You'll absorb fear, pain, trauma, grief, and uncertainty.

Even when you're off the clock, your patients stay with you.

This isn't the kind of job you "leave at the office."

2. You are always learning — and required to be.

The pace of medicine never slows.

Guidelines change.

Evidence evolves.

Your responsibilities expand.

You will forever live in a state of "there's more to know."

Some people thrive here.

Others drown.

3. The documentation burden is real.

EHRs don't care how compassionate you are.

Insurance doesn't reward intuition.

Audits don't forgive shortcuts.

You must document thoroughly, accurately, and defensively — every day, every visit.

It can be draining.

4. Burnout is a real, structural threat.

NPs are often the shock absorbers of the healthcare system — more accessible than physicians, more available, more flexible. That visibility can lead to overwhelming patient loads, unrealistic expectations, and systemic pressure that wears on your body and spirit.

Boundaries aren't optional.

They're survival.

5. Scope, laws, and autonomy vary wildly.

One state may treat you as a full autonomous provider.

Another may restrict your practice.

Your autonomy can change simply by crossing a state line — or switching employers.

You need to know your scope cold and protect it fiercely.

6. You will make mistakes — and you must learn to recover from them.

Not catastrophic mistakes, not daily mistakes — but human mistakes. And you will need to assume responsibility, reflect honestly, and keep practicing with courage.

This is a profession that demands humility.

• • •

Who Thrives Here — And Who Struggles

People who thrive as Nurse Practitioners tend to be:

- Curious and unafraid of lifelong learning
- Empathetic but not absorbent
- Calm under pressure
- Systematic thinkers
- Good communicators
- Conflict-tolerant
- Comfortable with uncertainty
- Advocates by instinct and habit
- Deeply aligned with the "why" of healthcare

People who struggle in this role tend to be:

- Overly perfectionistic
- Conflict-avoidant
- Uncomfortable making decisions
- Fearful of ambiguity
- Easily depleted by emotional labor
- Resistant to documentation
- Drawn to the role for the wrong reasons (income, title, external validation)

This isn't judgment.

This is alignment.

• • •

The Takeaway — And the Truth That Matters Most

The NP role is not "easier than medicine" or "a faster way to be a provider."

It is its own discipline.

Its own identity.

Its own calling.

It demands clinical rigor, emotional stamina, sharp judgment, soft listening, and fierce advocacy. It requires a brain trained in diagnostics and a heart trained in humanity.

But if you read this chapter and something inside you whispered

yes... this feels like me —

then keep going.

You might be built for this.

And if something whispered

I'm not sure —

that's not a red flag; it's good data.

This book will help you sort clarity from noise — so when you finally step into your first exam room as an NP, it won't feel like a costume.

It will feel like coming home.

Chapter 49

Student Success Stories

Student Success Stories: Six Journeys Into the Nurse Practitioner Profession.

1. MARIA — THE CAREER-CHANGER WHO STARTED OVER AT 42

Genre: Transformational Drama

Setting: 6:12 AM, a Honda Accord in a corporate parking lot

Maria's alarm always went off at 5:17 AM — a strange time she'd chosen years ago because it made her feel "slightly different" than the rest of the world. A tiny rebellion. But on this Tuesday, the rebel was tired. She sat in her car gripping a travel mug of coffee that tasted faintly like metal and resignation.

She watched other employees make the familiar walk from car door to glass-entrance. Everyone carried the same laptop bag. The same neutral expression. The same hollow Wednesday energy, even though it was Tuesday.

She whispered to her own reflection:

"I can't do this anymore."

It wasn't dramatic — just a truth that finally surfaced.

She went home, opened her laptop, and typed:

"Meaningful careers for adults starting over."

The algorithm did what algorithms do: it changed her life.

She landed on a forum thread about Nurse Practitioners. She read stories at midnight. She cried. She found herself imagining scrubs hanging on her closet door, textbooks with neon sticky notes, a badge that actually meant something.

The next month she enrolled in community college A&P.

She was terrified.

She was twice the age of everyone.

She sat next to a kid named Brayden who wore Crocs decorated with little plastic sushi charms.

She whispered to herself again:

"It's okay to begin."

Classes became a kind of rebirth. The first time she palpated a classmate's radial pulse during vitals lab, her chest tightened—not with anxiety, but with awe. Human connection. Purpose. Something she hadn't felt in years.

NP school wasn't easy. She studied in hospital cafeterias between clinical shifts, packed hummus and baby carrots like a monk, whispered pharmacology terms while folding laundry.

But graduation day?

She walked across that stage feeling like she'd returned to her real life.

Now, as a Family Nurse Practitioner, Maria is known for her presence. Her calm voice. Her eyes that never rush. Her 42-year-old rebirth gave her something younger students didn't have: perspective.

She tells new grads,

"Life doesn't start when you're young. Life starts when you decide to live it."

2. LUIS — THE FIRST-GENERATION STUDENT WHO REFUSED TO QUIT

Genre: Grit & Triumph

Setting: A cramped kitchen table, 11:58 PM, one flickering overhead bulb

Luis learned to translate before he learned long division.

At eight years old he stood between his mother and the doctor, converting Spanish trembling into English clarity. He did the same for his father's workers comp appointments, his aunt's diabetes follow-ups, his neighbor's ER visit after slicing a finger on a mandolin slicer.

He grew up understanding the power of a medical voice.

In nursing school, he struggled. He worked nights stocking shelves at Target. He slept in two-hour shifts. He failed his first med-surg exam. His advisor said gently,

"Healthcare is hard. It isn't for everyone."

But Luis had seen harder things.

He taped flashcards to the wall above his bed — red for pharm, blue for patho, yellow for cardio. He repeated terms until he could recite them while half-asleep. He built a study group of misfits: Jordan the former mechanic, Priya the bio major who hated blood, Andre who only studied after his son was asleep.

He graduated nursing school with a GPA that wasn't impressive but was *earned.*

NP school brought the magic.

Something clicked.

Suddenly, patients weren't just cases — they were stories he'd known his whole life. His bilingual skills became a superpower. His cultural intuition became clinical intuition.

On his first day as an NP, a patient's grandmother clasped his hands and said in Spanish,

"You speak the language of my heart."

Luis went home that night, placed his NP badge on the counter, and cried — not from exhaustion, but from arrival.

3. TAYLOR — THE ICU NURSE WHO WANTED TO THINK, NOT JUST FOLLOW ORDERS

Genre: Medical Thriller to Personal Breakthrough

Setting: ICU break room, 3:07 AM, stale donuts and fluorescent lights

Taylor loved the ICU. Loved the adrenaline, the machinery, the codes, the team that moved like a single organism with twelve arms. But after years at the bedside, a quiet resentment grew — not toward anyone, but the feeling of being trapped behind invisible glass.

She knew what each vent wave meant. She knew when a patient was about to tank before the monitor did. She knew the why beneath the what.

But she couldn't decide. She could only carry out decisions.

She told a coworker during a 3 AM break:

"I don't want to just execute the plan. I want to create it."

She enrolled in an Acute Care NP program and worked 3x12s. She studied on meal breaks with cold coffee and graham crackers. She watched pharmacology lectures on treadmill walks. She learned she could cry and review HFrEF guidelines simultaneously.

The first time her clinical preceptor said,

"Okay Taylor, what's your plan?"

— she froze. Then she breathed. Then she spoke.

Her voice trembled, but her reasoning didn't.

Now she works in the same ICU, but with a different badge and a different burden.

She rounds with the team.

She leads decisions.

She is the calm voice in the storm she once sprinted through.

Taylor says becoming an NP wasn't about climbing — it was about finally practicing medicine at the level she was built for.

4. JASMINE — THE SINGLE MOM WHO BUILT A NEW LIFE ONE CLASS AT A TIME

Genre: Heartfelt Drama

Setting: 8:42 PM, kitchen table, crayons everywhere, chicken nuggets cooling

Jasmine had her son at nineteen. She became a CNA because it was the quickest path to income. She worked double shifts, lifted patients twice her size, smiled through exhaustion that lived under her skin.

She carried a secret dream:

"I want to be the one explaining the plan — not the one transporting the chart."

She taped a sticky note inside her wallet:

NP by 30.

Life wasn't linear. She took *one* course a semester. Community college. Nights. Online discussion posts typed with one hand while holding a sleeping toddler with the other.

Biology. A&P. Micro. Statistics. Human growth and development.

Friends went out on weekends. Jasmine meal-prepped.

Friends posted vacation pics. Jasmine posted textbook stacks.

When she got into NP school, she cried so hard she scared her son.

“Mommy, what’s wrong?”

“Nothing,” she laughed through tears. “Absolutely nothing.”

She finished her program at exactly 30.

She crossed the stage holding her son’s hand.

The sticky note is framed on her office wall today.

Jasmine works in pediatric primary care — fitting, because she’s been raising two things her whole adult life: a child, and herself.

5. ETHAN — THE MILITARY MEDIC WHO LOST HIS IDENTITY AND FOUND IT AGAIN

Genre: Redemption Arc

Setting: VA Hospital parking lot, 4:55 PM, late autumn sunlight**

Ethan spent eight years as an Army medic. Deployment taught him how to make impossible decisions in impossible moments. He sutured in the dark. He stabilized chest wounds under helicopter blades. He treated dehydration, heat stroke, shrapnel wounds, and broken spirits.

Coming home was harder than deployment.

Civilian employers said,

"You don't have the right experience."

He wanted to scream, *"I kept people alive in a war zone."*

His identity crumpled.

His résumé felt like a lie.

He drifted between jobs, feeling invisible in a world that moved slower than his body was used to.

A mentor told him,

"You don't need to start over. You need the credential that proves what you already know."

NP school felt like resurfacing. Academic writing was torture. APA format nearly destroyed him. But in clinical?

He was brilliant.

He saw patterns before others spoke them.

He anticipated decline before monitors hinted at trouble.

His preceptor whispered to faculty,

"This one's built for emergency care."

Now Ethan is an Emergency NP.

His patients don't know his past.

They just know they feel safe around him.

He says being an NP is "the closest thing to purpose I've felt since active duty."

. . .

6. SOPHIE — THE BURNED-OUT STAR WHO REDISCOVERED HER HEART

Genre: Emotional Drama

Setting: 10:17 PM, car parked outside her apartment, engine still running**

Sophie was the golden child of her BSN program. Preceptor by 28. Charge nurse by 29. Committee lead by 30.

And absolutely falling apart by 31.

She loved nursing — but hated what it had become for her: constant chaos, pressure to chart faster, guilt about rushed care, and a deep ache that felt like grief. She'd sit in her car after her shift with her badge still around her neck, too tired to put the keys in the ignition.

Her therapist asked:

"Do you hate nursing, or do you hate not being able to nurse the way you want?"

That question peeled her open.

She shadowed an NP in women's health and cried in her car afterward — not because she was sad, but because she finally saw a version of nursing where care and thoughtfulness wasn't optional; it was woven into the role.

NP school became her reset button.

New pace.

New purpose.

New version of herself.

Today Sophie works in women's health as an NP, guiding adolescents, new mothers, and women navigating life transitions. She says:

"I didn't leave nursing. I came home to it."

About the Author

Mason Preddy brings **more than two and a half decades of experience in clinical healthcare recruitment, retention, and workforce strategy** to the ScrubTales™ series. Over the course of his career, he has worked closely with nurses, nurse practitioners, physicians, educators, executives, and healthcare systems across the country—supporting hiring decisions, career transitions, burnout recovery, and long-term workforce sustainability.

His background spans frontline clinical recruitment, leadership advisory work, workforce planning, and retention strategy, giving him a rare inside view of how healthcare careers actually unfold—not just in job descriptions, but in lived reality. Through this work, Mason has seen firsthand why some clinicians thrive in advanced practice roles while others quietly struggle, even when they are highly capable and well-trained.

Mason is the writer of ***What Color Are Your Scrubs?***, a comprehensive, alignment-first guide to healthcare careers, and the creator of the decision frameworks that anchor the ScrubTales™ series, including **PACES™**, **CARESET™**, and the **SCRUB*fit*™ Role Fit Index**. These tools are designed to help healthcare professionals evaluate fit, sustainability, and identity alignment before committing years of education, debt, and emotional energy to a role.

As the founder of Mason Maison™ Publishing, Mason writes with a singular focus: helping healthcare professionals make clearer, more honest career decisions grounded in who they are, how they are wired, and what they need to thrive over the long term.

Also by Mason Maison™ Publishing

Chapter 50

SCRUBfit™ Role Fit Index (RFI)

SCRUB*fit*™ Role Fit Index (RFI) — Nurse Practitioner

Are You Aligned With the Nurse Practitioner Path?

Wondering if becoming a **Nurse Practitioner (NP)** aligns with who you are — not just what you can do?

This short 15-question self-assessment is designed to help you gauge whether your personality, work preferences, and values fit the rhythm of advanced practice nursing.

It's not a test of skill. It's a mirror of alignment.

Take a breath, answer honestly, and trust what resonates.

Instructions

For each statement below, rate how true it feels for you on a scale of **1–10**:

1 = Not at all true **10 = Completely true**

Jot your number beside each statement, then total your points at the end.

Questions

1 I feel energized when I'm trusted to make independent clinical decisions.

2 I enjoy blending science and compassion to guide patients toward better outcomes.

3 I'm confident balancing autonomy with accountability in patient care.

4 I find fulfillment in developing long-term relationships with patients and families.

5 I enjoy translating complex medical information into language anyone can understand.

6 I'm comfortable managing uncertainty and adapting as new evidence emerges.

7 I see healthcare as both a profession and a platform for education and advocacy.

8 I feel calm and capable during high-stakes decision-making.

9 I'm drawn to both leadership and collaboration — guiding others while still learning.

10 I can manage emotional weight without losing empathy.

11 I find joy in mentoring students, residents, or newer nurses.

12 I prefer leading care plans over following prescriptive routines.

13 I stay motivated by improving systems, not just solving single problems.

14 I feel a strong pull toward prevention, education, and lifelong learning.

15 I see the Nurse Practitioner role as a natural evolution of my purpose in healthcare.

Scoring Guide

Add up your scores for all 15 questions.

Your total will fall within one of three alignment zones:

Total Points

Alignment Zone

Interpretation

120–150

High Alignment

You're deeply attuned to advanced practice. Your drive for autonomy, empathy, and lifelong learning aligns beautifully with the Nurse Practitioner path. This role may be your natural next chapter.

90–119

Partial Alignment

You share many NP traits — critical thinking, empathy, and independence — but may prefer another **SCRUB*fit*™** category (like **The Vital Link** or **The Compassion Corps**). Explore before committing to grad school.

Below 90

Misalignment Zone

You may thrive better in another area of healthcare. That's not failure — it's self-awareness. Consider exploring other roles that better reflect your rhythm and resilience.

Reflection Prompt

Circle or underline three statements that made you pause — the ones that felt truest *or* most uncertain.

Those moments reveal your alignment story.

Ask yourself:

"What do these answers tell me about the kind of healer I want to be?"

As you reflected on these questions, you may have noticed patterns — the kinds of moments that energize you, the responsibilities you welcome, and the environments where you think most clearly.

Those patterns show up across healthcare in different ways. In the next section, you'll meet the **SCRUB*fits*™** — guides who represent different styles of working, leading, caring, and contributing.

You may recognize yourself in one or two of them. That recognition isn't a label. It's a clue.

Next Step

For a deeper, personalized look at your healthcare alignment across all 21 **SCRUB*fit*™** roles, take the complete **SCRUB*fit*™**

Healthcare Career Assessment — available at masonmaison.pub.

Use **Promo Code: smart** for **25% off** your assessment.

Because the opposite of alignment isn't failure — it's a miserable life.

Choose alignment. Thrive in your calling.

Love every minute of your career.

Chapter 51

About the SCRUBfit™ Role Fit Index (RFI)

About the SCRUB*fit*™ Role Fit Index (RFI)

The **SCRUB*fit*™ Role Fit Index (RFI)** was designed to answer a simple but often overlooked question in healthcare careers:

Does this role fit how I'm wired — not just what I can do?

Most career decisions in healthcare are made based on credentials, job availability, or external expectations. The RFI shifts the focus inward, toward alignment between identity, environment, and day-to-day work demands.

How the RFI Was Designed

The RFI is grounded in patterns observed across thousands of healthcare careers. Its questions reflect recurring themes that influence long-term satisfaction and sustainability, including:

- Preference for autonomy versus structure
- Comfort with uncertainty and responsibility

- Desire for continuity versus episodic interaction
- Tolerance for emotional weight
- Interest in leadership, education, or systems change

Rather than measuring skill or readiness, the RFI looks at **energy patterns** — what tends to energize you over time, and what consistently drains you.

What the RFI Tells You

The RFI offers a snapshot of how well a specific role aligns with your current preferences, values, and work style. It can help you:

- Anticipate sources of satisfaction or friction
- Clarify whether discomfort is developmental or structural
- Decide where exploration may be helpful
- Normalize curiosity about other roles without judgment

Your score reflects alignment *in this season*, not a permanent label.

What the RFI Does Not Tell You

The RFI does not measure intelligence, clinical competence, or potential.

It does not predict success, income, or status.

It does not tell you what you *should* do.

Many people succeed in roles that don't align with them — often at the cost of burnout. The RFI exists to surface that tension early, so choices can be made with awareness rather than endurance.

Using the RFI Wisely

A high RFI score doesn't mean you're obligated to pursue this role.

A lower score doesn't mean you should leave healthcare.

It simply means you have information.

Alignment is not about finding the "right" job once. It's about understanding yourself well enough to adjust, pivot, or explore thoughtfully over time.

That's the purpose of the RFI — and of this book.

Chapter 52

Good Bye For Now

The Never End™ — How to Use This Book Going Forward

This book is not a graduation speech. It's a reference system for the moments your career stops feeling simple.

Because Nurse Practitioner work doesn't break people loudly. It wears them down quietly — in the small, repeated collisions between responsibility and time, between what patients need and what the schedule allows, between your clinical judgment and the constraints you didn't agree to but now have to live inside. Most NPs don't wake up one morning and decide they're done. They wake up one morning and realize they've been carrying something too heavy for too long, and nobody handed them a map.

That's what this book is for.

You don't reread it front to back. You return to the chapter that matches the pressure you're under right now, the same way you'd return to a trusted protocol when the room gets tense. Use it the way high-functioning clinicians use tools: not because you don't know what to do, but because you refuse to make high-stakes decisions on guesswork, momentum, or emotional exhaustion.

When you're interviewing and trying to tell the difference between a good offer and a good trap, come back to the hiring sequence and **Terms of Care™** and read with a sharper eye. When your documentation starts following you home and you're quietly normalizing it, come back to the boundaries sections and recalibrate before that becomes your baseline. When you can't tell whether you're tired or misaligned, return to **PACES™ & CARESET™** and separate "me" from "the conditions," because those are not the same thing — and confusing them ruins careers.

If you're early in practice, this book helps you avoid the most common mistake new NPs make: believing struggle is proof you're not cut out for it. In reality, struggle is often proof that the onboarding is thin, the expectations are unspoken, or the environment is misaligned — and your job is to name that early, not endure it until it becomes identity. If you're years in, this book helps you stop drifting. It helps you choose your next move intentionally — specialty shifts, role redesign, leadership, entrepreneurship, or an exit ramp that preserves your health and your dignity.

This is the promise of The Never End™: you will not outgrow the need to re-check alignment. You will outgrow certain seasons, certain settings, certain versions of yourself — and that is not failure. That is evolution. Your career will ask you, again and again, to renegotiate what you will carry, what you will protect, and what you will no longer pretend is sustainable.

Return to this book any time you feel the early warning signs: dread that doesn't match the job on paper, irritability that feels unlike you, chronic exhaustion that rest doesn't fix, or the slow disappearance of joy. Those aren't character flaws. They're data. And you deserve to treat them like data — early, honestly, and without shame.

Alignment is not a one-time decision you make before school. It is a professional practice you return to, especially when life changes, leadership changes, the patient load changes, the laws change, or you change.

So keep this book close. Not as motivation. As a map.

Because the goal isn't to become an NP and survive it.

The goal is to become an NP and stay whole.

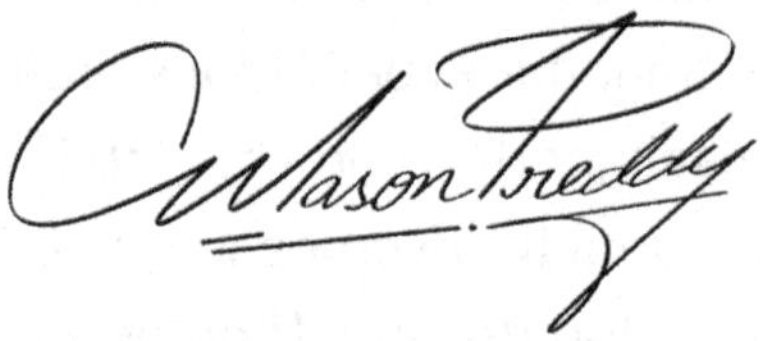

Chapter 53

Glossary

Made in the USA
Monee, IL
05 November 2026

67911922R00197